PIONEERS OF MEDICINE
WITHOUT A
NOBEL PRIZE

PIONEERS OF MEDICINE
WITHOUT A
NOBEL PRIZE

Editor

Gilbert Thompson

Imperial College London, UK

Imperial College Press

ICP

Published by

Imperial College Press
57 Shelton Street
Covent Garden
London WC2H 9HE

Distributed by

World Scientific Publishing Co. Pte. Ltd.
5 Toh Tuck Link, Singapore 596224
USA office: 27 Warren Street, Suite 401-402, Hackensack, NJ 07601
UK office: 57 Shelton Street, Covent Garden, London WC2H 9HE

Library of Congress Control Number: **2013957214**

British Library Cataloguing-in-Publication Data
A catalogue record for this book is available from the British Library.

PIONEERS OF MEDICINE WITHOUT A NOBEL PRIZE

ISBN 978-1-78326-383-7
ISBN 978-1-78326-384-4 (pbk)

Typeset by Stallion Press
Email: enquiries@stallionpress.com

Printed in Singapore by Mainland Press Pte Ltd.

CONTENTS

FOREWORD

I once asked a newly immigrant New York taxi driver about his family history. He was simply not interested — he was engaged in the struggle of finding a new life for his family in a new country. Family history, he averred dismissively, was for the established, the comfortable and the wealthy. So it is with medical history. Young doctors are far more interested in the contemporary science and practice of medicine than in learning how we reached our present understanding of the mechanisms of health and disease.

I remember being amazed, when researching the introduction to my PhD thesis, to discover that much of what I thought was new and undiscovered about the complement system had been characterised first by researchers in the 1920s and 1930s, working on the serological detection of trypanosomes in Africa. This made me realise the importance of studying the past as an integral part of researching for the future.

Similarly, it was one man's adventure story of a discovery, *The Double Helix* by James Watson, that inspired me and many of my generation to become medical researchers, in the same way that *Microbe Hunters* by Paul Kruiff inspired earlier generations.

Pioneers of Medicine without a Nobel Prize is a book for the young written by the not-so-young. It is an engaging series of accounts of adventures in the clinic and the laboratory by a group of scientists, some well-known and others barely remembered. These stories of discovery, accompanied by thumbnail biographies of their protagonists, inspire and remind us of the origins of an important selection of the health advances made by medical researchers in the 20th century.

The title of this book, *Pioneers of Medicine without a Nobel Prize*, gives pause for thought. Is this a way to define these pioneers? It is not. The common denominator of these scientists, chosen mainly for having made important clinical contributions that improved public health and reduced suffering from diseases, is that they were dogged individualists who identified important questions for medical research and tackled them with sustained determination. I think that most of them would not define themselves in terms of a negative and nor should we.

It is an abiding problem of prizes that they add much more to the sum of human unhappiness than the converse — and the Nobel Prize is supreme in this achievement. Discovery has many parents. Almost without exception it builds on the work of others and is usually a product of teams of individuals. None of this is recognised by the Nobel Prizes. These reward no more than three people for each prize and have a history for Physiology or Medicine of being awarded far more often to basic rather than clinical discoveries.

Several of the stories in this book show the importance of 'ripeness of time', of a milieu in which important questions effectively 'declare themselves' and the technology is at the point at which it can be developed to provide the answers. Many of these discoveries did receive important prizes, Lasker Awards, Gairdner Awards, or the Japan Prize, but I suspect that a similar array could be assembled that did not win any prizes at all.

This book looks underneath the prizes — at the scientists, their work, their motivations and their backgrounds. Its message is that medical research is challenging, sometimes frustrating, often fun and brings that greatest prize of all, a major contribution to the well-being of humans and other species.

Mark Walport,
May 2013.

PREFACE

Know ye not that they which run in a race run all,
but one receiveth the prize?
I Corinthians 9:24

Some of the outstanding scientists and physicians to receive the Nobel Prize in Physiology or Medicine were depicted recently in *Nobel Prizes that Changed Medicine*. This book is the sequel and describes an equally remarkable group of individuals who, despite the importance of their discoveries for Medicine, have not received the Nobel Prize. Most of them never will because they are deceased and it is not awarded posthumously. However, some of those still living may yet succeed — the oldest winner, Peyton Rous, was 87 at the time of his award.

Many of the individuals who feature in this volume have been recipients of a Lasker Award, often regarded as America's equivalent of the Nobel Prize. The aptness of this analogy is illustrated by the fact that almost half of the Nobel laureates in Physiology or Medicine since World War II had already won Lasker Awards. The latter were inaugurated in 1946 by Albert and Mary Lasker, now both dead, but like Alfred Nobel their legacy of rewarding excellence lives on after them. It is striking that nearly all of the Nobel Prize winners featured in *Nobel Prizes that changed Medicine* who had previously won a Lasker were given a Basic Medical Research Award whereas most of the scientists in *Pioneers of Medicine without a Nobel Prize* who won a Lasker received a Clinical Medical Research Award; this suggests that clinical or applied research is regarded less highly than basic research by the Nobel Assembly. The current emphasis on translational

ix

research, deplored recently by JS Goldstein and MS Brown,[1] militates against Nobel Prize-winning scientists of the future having a clinical background — as they did and as did the seven other Nobel laureates who trained at the National Institutes of Health (NIH) between 1964 and 1972.

Despite the caveats, inclusion in this book is emphatically not an indication of second class status, of not being quite good enough to get a Nobel Prize. Comparisons are invidious but arguably the discovery of statins has prolonged just as many lives, probably more, than did the introduction of penicillin. In a similar vein, it is debatable whether the prevention of Rh disease in neonates is any less important than discovering the cure for pernicious anaemia. The fact is that there are simply not enough Nobel Prizes to reward all those who have made major discoveries since they were inaugurated in 1901. The Prize in Physiology or Medicine is limited to a maximum of three laureates annually and an *embarras de richesses* of outstanding candidates means that hard and difficult choices have to be made every year in Stockholm.

This dilemma might be resolved if the Physiology and Medicine components of the Prize were treated as separate awards, thereby doubling the number of potential recipients. Thus the Prize in Physiology would be for basic scientific discoveries whereas the Prize in Medicine would be reserved for discoveries in applied or clinical science.

The physicians, surgeons and scientists described in the following chapters have individually and collectively made enormous contributions to the prevention, diagnosis and treatment of disease. Their discoveries span a variety of scientific disciplines ranging from epidemiology to preventive medicine, from nephrology to cardiac surgery, and from experimental haematology to molecular genetics. Whether they should have been awarded the Nobel Prize and why they haven't been remains a matter of conjecture and is the stuff of this book.

Gilbert Thompson

---

[1] A golden era of Nobel laureates, *Science* 2012; 338: 1033–1034.

ACKNOWLEDGEMENTS

I am most grateful to all the authors who took the time and effort to write chapters for this book, especially those who had previously contributed to its precursor, *Nobel Prizes that changed Medicine*. I apologise to them for piling Pelion upon Ossa! This analogy is equally applicable to Sir Mark Walport, who kindly wrote the Foreword while in the throes of relinquishing the Directorship of the Wellcome Trust to become Chief Scientific Advisor to HM Government. My thanks go to him and also to Elizabeth Manson, who assisted with the indexing, and again to Jacqueline Downs and her colleagues at Imperial College Press for their help and guidance during the publication process. Lastly, I wish to acknowledge the help and advice I received when planning the contents of this book from the distinguished clinical scientist and historian, Sir Christopher Booth, and from his and my erstwhile colleague, Professor Graham Neale, both recently deceased.

CONTRIBUTORS

Bhavna Batohi, MB, BS, BSc.
Research Fellow
Department of Radiology, King's College Hospital, London.

Karel A. Dicke, MD, PhD.
Oncology Specialist
Hematology/Oncology, BMT-unit, Arlington Cancer Center,
Arlington, Texas.

David J. Galton, MD, FRCP, DSc.
Professor of Human Metabolism
Department of Genetics & Metabolism, Wolfson Institute
of Medicine, St. Bartholmew's Hospital, London.

Marc G. Ghany, MD, MHSc.
Staff Physician
Liver Diseases Branch, National Institutes of Diabetes,
Digestive and Kidney Diseases, National Institutes of Health,
Bethesda, Maryland.

Max Lab, MD, PhD.
Professor Emeritus and Senior Research Investigator
National Heart & Lung Institute, Imperial College, London.

Peter A. Leggat, MD, PhD, DrPH.
Director, Anton Breinl Centre
James Cook University, Townsville, Queensland.

Hiroshi Mabuchi, MD.
Research Professor
Kanazawa University, Kanazawa.

David Marais, MB ChB (UCT), FCP (SA).
Professor of Chemical Pathology
University of Cape Town, Cape Town.

Chris J. J. Mulder, MD, PhD.
Professor of Gastroenterology
VU University Medical Center, Amsterdam.

Tony Seed, BM, PhD, FRCP.
Emeritus Professor of Medicine
National Heart and Lung Institute, Imperial College,
Charing Cross Hospital, London.

Leonard B. Seeff, MD.
Consultant in Hepatology
The Hill Group, Bethesda, Maryland and the U.S. Food & Drug
Administration, Silver Spring, Maryland.

Paul S. Sidhu, MRCP, FRCR.
Professor of Imaging Sciences
Department of Radiology, King's College Hospital, London.

Derek R. Smith, PhD, MPH.
Professor of Environmental and Occupational Health
University of Newcastle, Ourimbah, New South Wales.

Joe Sornberger
Author, *Dreams and Due Diligence*, University of Toronto Press
Ottawa, Ontario.

Anne Soutar, PhD.
Professor of Molecular Genetics
MRC Clinical Sciences Centre, Imperial College, Hammersmith
Hospital, London.

Daniel Steinberg, MD, PhD.
Professor of Medicine Emeritus
University of California San Diego, La Jolla, California.

Gilbert Thompson, MD, FRCP.
Emeritus Professor of Clinical Lipidology
Metabolic Medicine, Imperial College,
Hammersmith Hospital, London.

John Turney, MA, MD, FRCP.
Retired Renal Physician
Centre for History of Science Technology and Medicine,
University of Manchester, Manchester.

Sir Mark Walport, FRS, FMedSci.
Chief Scientific Advisor to HM Government
Government Office for Science, London.

Sir David J. Weatherall, FRS, FRCP.
Regius Professor of Medicine Emeritus
Weatherall Institute of Molecular Medicine,
University of Oxford, Oxford.

Stephen Westaby, MS, PhD, FRCS.
Professor of Cardiothoracic Surgery
Department of Cardiothoracic Surgery,
John Radcliffe Hospital, Oxford.

Chapter 1

ARCHIBALD E. GARROD: THE FOUNDING FATHER OF BIOCHEMICAL GENETICS

David J. Galton

1.1 Introduction

In the 1890s Archibald Garrod, a physician at St. Bartholomew's Hospital in London, embarked on a seemingly trivial project to study the occurrence of unusual urinary pigments, a topic derided by his colleagues as 'playing around with urine'. Admittedly, the major interest of the 19th century was to understand the nature of infectious disease, led by such luminaries as Pasteur, Koch, Erhlich and Widal. But despite active discouragement from colleagues, Garrod produced data that initiated three new fields of study and generated two insights that have proved equally fruitful. The ability to foresee and correctly formulate hitherto unrecognized problems and provide solutions that open up new areas of knowledge is a gift requiring rare genius, which Garrod had in full measure. His major research achievements are outlined below.

1.1.1 *Discovery of the inborn errors of metabolism (1901)*

Garrod found that the cause of alkaptonuria (black urine trait)[1,2] was a defective enzyme on the catabolic pathway of phenylalanine. The defect occurs at the reaction splitting the benzene ring of homogentisic acid to form maleylacetoacetic acid. The catabolism of homogentisic acid is therefore blocked and consequently it is excreted at high concentrations in the urine. Here it polymerises to form dark pigments similar to the family of melanins.[3] Garrod termed the condition an 'inborn error of metabolism' and in 1908 he described three other conditions that could arise on a similar basis: pentosuria, cystinuria and albinism.[4] Subsequent work has shown that Garrod was correct in regarding pentosuria and albinism as being due to enzyme defects, whereas cystinuria is more complicated, some types being due to defects in a heteromeric amino acid transporter in the renal tubules. The genomic loci of Garrod's four inborn errors have now been mapped, the genes cloned, the mutations identified and annotated and the relevant gene products isolated and characterized.[5]

1.1.2 First application of Mendelian genetics to clinical medicine (1902)

In Garrod's study of the segregation of alkaptonuria in the offspring of first cousin marriages he observed approximate Mendelian ratios for recessive inheritance in affected versus total family members (Table 1.1). The prevalent view at the time, originating from the work of Charles Darwin and formulated in detail by Garrod's contemporary, Karl Pearson (1857–1936), was that inherited variation was continuous. Pearson was the leading proponent for the Biometricians in the debate with the Mendelians (led by William Bateson) in the early part of the 20th century. The Biometricians called

Table 1.1.   Data from Garrod's publication in the *Lancet* in 1902 showing the large proportion of alkaptonurics who are the offspring of first cousin marriages.[3]

Family no.	Family members	Alkaptonurics
1	14	4
2	4	3
3	5	2
4	1	1
5	8	1
6	4	1
Total	36	12

it blending inheritance, exemplified by the skin colour of offspring from black-white marriages. In Garrod's studies inheritance appeared to be discontinuous, that is family members either excreted homogentisic acid at high concentrations in their urine or did not; there were no intermediate signs of blending. So these observations better fitted the Mendelian recessive model of discontinuity.

Garrod's findings were first published by the Evolution Committee of the Royal Society during 1901 under the aegis of Bateson.[6] In 1902 Garrod published the results of his studies on first cousin marriages in the *Lancet* and these data strongly suggested that Mendel's model of inheritance applied also to man: 'It has recently been pointed out by Bateson that the law of heredity discovered by Mendel offers a reasonable account of such phenomena.'[3]

Garrod went further than Mendel in his *Lancet* paper[3] by suggesting that the accumulation of homogentisic acid might be due to a block in the normal catabolic pathway for disposal of this metabolite. Since these metabolic reactions are under the control of enzymes it is possible that alkaptonurics were making a defective enzyme that was unable to break down homogentisic acid.[7] This gave Mendel's factors of inheritance (called *merkmal* by Mendel) a biochemical function, namely making proteins such as enzymes to regulate the chemical reactions in cells.

Garrod had collected similar information for albino families. This inherited condition is due to a failure to produce pigments of the melanin group in the skin. When he studied the incidence of albinism in such families he found the same numerical ratios for affected individuals, about 1:3, as he found for alkaptonuria. He had studied a third condition, cystinuria, and again the pattern of inheritance in affected families fitted the Mendelian model. Garrod concluded that the laws of heredity as discovered by Mendel offered the best explanation for his own observations.[7]

1.1.3 *First recognition of 'gene'–enzyme relationships (1902)*

Three other scientists, all botanists (Carl Correns,[8] 1864–1933; Hugo de Vries,[9] 1848–1935 and Erich von Tschermak,[10] 1871–1962) working at major European universities, replicated Mendel's studies of recessive inheritance at the start of the 20th century. But Garrod went a step further because he studied the chemistry underlying the pigmented urine in alkaptonuria, whereas the three botanists, also studying pigmentation of petals and seed coats (amongst other traits), had not done the basic biochemistry. Garrod concluded from his studies that 'the splitting of the benzene ring in normal metabolism is the work of a specific enzyme that in congenital alkaptonuria is wanting ...'.[4] This was the first recognition that Mendelian factors (the word 'gene' had not yet been coined) were related to enzymes, and led later to the 'one gene-one enzyme' hypothesis.[11]

Fifty years later George Beadle and Edward Tatum were awarded the Nobel Prize for the formulation of the 'one gene-one enzyme' hypothesis, mainly on work with mutants of the bread mould *Neurospora*. They generously acknowledged in their acceptance speech that, 'in this long and roundabout way, first in *Drosophila* and then in *Neurospora*, we had rediscovered what Garrod had seen so clearly so many years before. By now we knew of his work and were aware that we had added little if anything new in principle. We were working with a more favourable organism and were able to produce, almost at will, inborn errors of metabolism for almost any chemical reaction whose product we could supply through the medium; thus we were able to demonstrate that what Garrod had shown for a few genes and a few chemical reactions in man was true for many genes and many reactions in *Neurospora*' (Beadle, 1958 cited by Olby.)[12]

1.1.4 *First ideas on chemical individuality (1902)*

Garrod, from his study of alkaptonuria, suggested: 'May it not well be that there are other such chemical abnormalities that are attended by no obvious peculiarities and which could only be revealed by chemical analysis?'[3] He went on to propose that 'in alkaptonuria and other conditions mentioned we are dealing with individualities of metabolism and not with the results of morbid processes ... [T]hese are merely extreme examples of variation of chemical behaviour which are probably everywhere present in minor degrees ... [J]ust as no two individuals of a species are absolutely identical in bodily structure neither are their chemical processes carried out on exactly the same lines.' He suggested that: 'Individuals of a species do not conform to an absolutely rigid standard of metabolism but differ slightly in their chemistry as they do in their structure.'

We now know this to be true, taking the form of polymorphisms of enzymes, receptors, transporters and DNA sequences. Single amino-acid substitutions at one of several sites in a peptide chain are compatible with normal or near-normal function of that peptide. However, substitutions at active sites in the peptide can profoundly modify its function causing disease. Such disease is therefore just the tip of an iceberg of a number of minor individual variants or 'sports' as Garrod called them. Common structural variation of DNA sequences are now most likely to be the inherited liability factors that Garrod writes about in the Croonian Lectures.[13] His idea of chemical individuality reaches its fullest expression in the use of DNA 'fingerprints' as the best means of identifying a person.

1.1.5 *Inherited liability to metabolic disease (1908)*

Garrod's second insight was succinctly stated by him as follows: 'The liability to develop diabetes or gout is often inherited, but the diseases themselves are not inherited for they are not present at birth. … Quite unlike the above metabolic diseases are the course of the anomalies … which may be classed as the inborn errors of metabolism.'[13]

Garrod considered that there must be at least two types of inheritance: a Mendelian type for the inborn errors of metabolism and a non-Mendelian type for the liability to inherit conditions like diabetes, obesity or gout (his examples). Later he wrote a research monograph entitled *The Inborn Factors in Disease*.[14] He was struck by the differences in response of humans to various environmental insults such as infectious agents, foreign antigens and drugs. He attributed this to differences in people's constitution — that is their 'biochemical individuality'. He supposed that differences in inborn biochemical factors can determine how a person will respond to the *tubercle bacillus* or the malarial plasmodia in terms of disease severity.

But he did not elaborate on his truly perceptive remarks regarding the liability factors for metabolic disease.

Currently we understand reasonably well the biochemical and genetic basis for most of the inborn errors of metabolism. But we are still a long way from understanding how the inherited liability to disease operates.

1.2 Biography

The main features of Garrod's life are sketched in Table 1.2. Archibald (called Archie from childhood since the boy hated the name Archibald) was born in 1857, the youngest son of Sir Alfred Baring Garrod. Sir Alfred was an able and talented doctor whose main claim to fame was the important discovery that patients suffering from gout had raised levels of uric acid in their blood. It turned out to be a good diagnostic test to distinguish the disease from other joint disorders such as rheumatoid arthritis. He went on to specialize in rheumatic disease and the *rue Sir Alfred Garrod* in Aix-les-Bains in Southern France is named after him. This is because Sir Alfred stressed the value of taking the mineral waters there for the treatment of gouty arthritis and the Town Council considered that he was responsible for making a sojourn at Aix a standard treatment for gout. Sir Alfred was later appointed as Professor to King's College in the Strand but gave up the post at the age of 55 years to concentrate on his lucrative private practice. He was appointed as a Physician to the Queen in 1888 and died a wealthy man.

Table 1.2   Selected stages in Garrod's life.

1857	Born in London, UK.
1884	Qualifies at Bart's Hospital, London.
1892	Publishes on red-coloured urine; the haematoporphyrins.
1897	Studies patients with alkaptonuria.
1902	Publishes classic paper in Lancet[3] on the incidence of alkaptonuria.
1914	Enlists for First World War; posted to Malta. Three sons killed in War.
1919	Appointed Regius Professor of Physic, Oxford University.
1931	Publishes an essay: 'Inborn Factors in Disease.'[14]
1936	Dies of coronary thrombosis.

The Garrods had six children, four boys and two girls.[15] Archie was the fifth child and was recalled as a nice-looking and well-mannered young lad (Fig. 1.1). He went to a public school, Marlborough College, and then to Christchurch College, Oxford. He qualified in medicine in 1884 at St. Bartholomew's Hospital in London. This is one of the oldest and most distinguished hospitals in Europe, founded in 1123.

Garrod started working at St. Bartholomew's in 1885 (Fig. 1.2). On entering through the Smithfield Gate you did not appear to be in a hospital. There were stately London plane trees lining a beautiful inner square with an old fountain at its centre. The consultant's offices were located in a grand building in the North Wing where visitors were usually taken. Dr Garrod was often absent since he also worked at the Hospital for Sick Children at Great Ormond Street.

Garrod's studies on urinary pigments had far-reaching implications for human inheritance. The work would have progressed further had not the hospital authorities been particularly mean-spirited towards Garrod. They had not yet promoted him to the staff of the

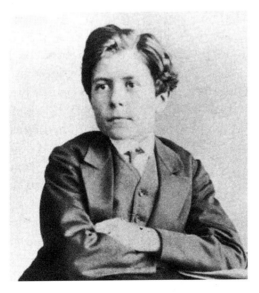

Fig. 1.1. Garrod as a teenager when at Marlborough College. (Reproduced with the permission of Professor Simon Garrod.)

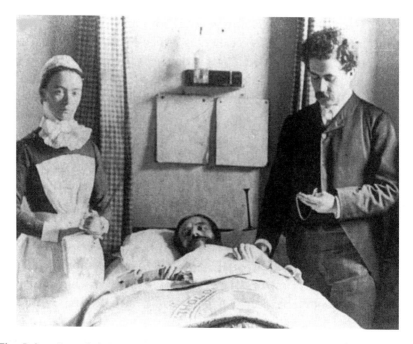

Fig. 1.2. Garrod doing a ward round at Bart's. (Reproduced with the permission of Professor Simon Garrod.)

hospital, he being only a chemical pathologist there. He had applied unsuccessfully for the post of Assistant Physician in 1887, again in 1893 and twice in 1895. However, when one of his colleagues was promoted to the rank of full Physician in 1902 he left a vacancy and this time Garrod was appointed as Assistant Physician at the age of 45. He was supported by 29 testimonials. Each letter could not have been more enthusiastic about his abilities and character, and all the writers showed their total embarrassment that Garrod had not been elected to the hospital staff sooner. It was disgraceful for a man with such analytical abilities and imagination to be so neglected. However, it had given him time to 'play around' with his urine specimens, as his colleagues described it, and make some fundamental progress in the study of human heredity.

In 1914 Garrod enlisted for World War I in the Royal Army Medical Corps.[16] The disastrous experiences of the British in the

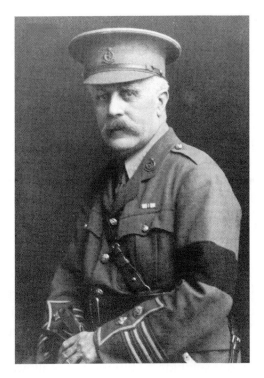

Fig. 1.3.   Colonel Garrod mourning the death of his three sons in World War I. (Reproduced with the permission of Professor Simon Garrod.)

Crimean War (1853–1856) were still very much in people's minds. The war had terrible consequences for Garrod. His three sons enlisted in 1914; two were killed in action and the third developed trench fever and died of pneumonia before the war ended (Fig. 1.3).

On his return to England in 1918 Garrod was appointed to the Regius Professorship of Medicine at the prestigious University of Oxford, his *alma mater*. One of the most interesting articles that Garrod published after the war was the essay entitled The Inborn Factors in Disease.[14] He also published numerous articles on such topics as the scientific spirit in medicine, medicine from the chemical standpoint, how to learn medicine and the debt of science to medicine (the Harveian Lecture of the Royal College of Physicians, London, 1924). He died in 1936 at the age of 78 from coronary thrombosis.

1.3   Research Methods

From Garrod's first publication on alkaptonuria in 1898 to his last in 1908 he used the simplest of methods.

1.3.1   Organic chemistry

He measured homogentisic acid in the urine of his subjects by precipitating it as the lead salt and then converting it into the ethyl ester by Meyer's method.[17] The resulting crystalline product had the melting point of ethyl homogentisate (120°C), so confirming its identity. His usual method was to heat the urine nearly to boiling and then add 5 gm of lead acetate to each 100 ml. of urine. The dense precipitate that formed was filtered off whilst the liquid was still hot and the clear yellow filtrate was allowed to cool. After a time lead homogentisate began to separate out in crystalline form and after 24 hours the crystals were filtered off, washed, dried and weighed. The free acid could be obtained by passing hydrogen sulphide through ether in which the powdered lead salt was suspended. When the solvent, freed from lead sulphide by filtration, was allowed to evaporate colourless crystals of homogentisic acid were left with a melting point of 146–147°C. In later studies he used the simpler method of Baumann[18] that depended on the reduction of silver nitrate in the presence of ammonia.

1.3.2   Pedigree analysis

Garrod linked his chemical analyses of urine to the study of pedigrees of alkaptonurics with no affected parents, to pedigrees with affected parents and to alkaptonurics who were the children of first cousin marriages. The latter pedigrees were analogous to the F2 generation of pea hybrids that Mendel had studied 50 years earlier.[19] Both of their studies showed a tendency to find a ratio of 1:3 for affected versus unaffected progeny for the trait under study.

1.3.3 *Feeding experiments*

Garrod conducted feeding experiments comparing proteins rich in phenylalanine, such as casein, with proteins such as egg albumin containing little of this amino acid. For unaffected relatives he never found homogentisic acid appearing in their urine after feeding casein; but when casein was fed to alkaptonurics the excretion of homogentisic acid increased in relation to the amount of casein consumed, suggesting a total catabolic block after that metabolite.[20]

1.4 Scope of Garrod's Impact

For most medical or scientific endeavours a single individual only makes a tiny contribution compared to the team effort of current colleagues and those before him; so any credit has to be shared with others. But Garrod almost single-handedly founded the subject of Biochemical Genetics. Like Mendel he was thinking so far ahead of his time that his work went largely unnoticed until enzymology matured[21,22] and became linked to genetics by the work of Beadle, Tatum and others.[23] The journal *Biochemical Genetics* was founded in 1967 to cover all the topics that Garrod initiated in his studies and to provide links between organic chemistry, metabolism and genetics.

1.4.1 *Inborn errors of metabolism*

Very few scientists have a learned society named after their discoveries, but Garrod was one of them. The Society for the Study of Inborn Errors of Metabolism (SSIEM for short) was founded in 1963 to promote exchange of ideas for people studying inherited metabolic disorders. The current members call themselves Garrodians and number well over 1,000, coming from more than 60 different countries. The Society arranges annual scientific meetings and publishes its affiliated *Journal of Inherited Metabolic Disease* (JIMD).

The origin of the SSIEM started with an informal meeting held at the Manchester Royal Infirmary in 1962 when an enthusiastic group of biochemists and paediatricians met to discuss phenylketonuria. The following year the same group held a symposium in Sheffield entitled 'Neurometabolic disorders in childhood'. The society was formally constituted in October 1963 and the first annual symposium was held in Liverpool in 1964 on the topic 'Biochemical approaches to mental handicap in children'.

Thereafter the topics of the SSIEM developed steadily[24] and the first symposium to be held outside Britain was at Zurich in 1968. One of the most important achievements of the SSIEM is its *Journal of Inherited Metabolic Disease* launched in 1978. All the symposia of the SSIEM have been published in the journal as well as reviews on topics in the field of inborn errors.

On 5 September 2008, more than 1,000 delegates of the SSIEM from around the world gathered in Lisbon to celebrate the life and work of Archibald Garrod.[25] This event was to mark the centenary of the publication in 1908 of his classic text *The Croonian Lectures on Inborn Errors of Metabolism*.[26] 'Garrod Day' was held in Lisbon and opened with a speech from the Portuguese Minister of Science and Culture, followed by speakers from North America, Germany and England. They included Leon Rosenberg from Princeton, Charles Scriver from McGill University, Montreal, Johannes Zschoke from Heidelberg University, Germany and William Gahl from the National Institutes of Health, US.

Garrod had postulated four conditions to be due to inherited metabolic defects; alkaptonuria, pentosuria and albinism are due to enzyme defects, whereas cystinuria in most cases turns out to be a transporter defect. We now know there are more than 8,000 such inborn errors. The 1972 edition of *Metabolic Basis of Inherited Disease*[27] describes about 1,000 disorders due to mutations in enzymes, hormones, receptors, transporters and structural proteins. The volume contains 1,725 pages with approximately 90 authors in 12 sections. When the book was reissued in 2000 as *The Metabolic and Molecular Basis of Inherited Disease* under the chief editorship of Charles R Scriver[28] it had enlarged to four volumes with 255 sections, 6,338 pages and more than 500 authors. It now has to be continuously expanded online as new information accumulates. Most scientific discoveries are after about 100 years just taken for granted, having become part of the accepted corpus of knowledge; but not Garrod's, which continually need to be updated.

Many therapeutic avenues have developed as a result of Garrod's early work. These include neonatal screening for the inborn errors, such as phenylketonuria; institution of appropriate diets; and the use of drug therapy to inhibit reactions before the metabolic defect to reduce the accumulation of the harmful metabolite. For example, Nitisinone inhibits the enzymatic step on the catabolic pathway of phenylalanine before the production of homogentisic acid and can reduce the metabolite load of the acid in the body by up to 95%.[29] Nitisinone reduces homogentisic acid excretion in urine from about 4 g/d to 0.2 g/d (normal < 0.03 g/d). As expected, plasma tyrosine concentration rises by about ten-fold but with no obvious ill-effects. Nitisinone is well tolerated; and although in trials it failed in its primary endpoint of increased joint movements, improvement of symptoms in some patients with established arthropathy was observed.

1.4.2 *Mutation research*

Since Garrod first detected that an enzyme was 'wanting' on the catabolic pathway of phenylalanine the subject has grown to enormous proportions. Garrod's feeding experiments showed an almost complete block in the enzyme splitting the benzene ring of homogentisic acid. Thus the ratio of homogentisic acid excreted in the urine to the amount of protein consumed was fairly constant.[20]

Identifying the nature of such mutant proteins can now explain the pathogenesis of thousands of human disorders. Furthermore it can illuminate the function of a particular protein *in vivo* much more convincingly than doing transgenic, knockout or knockdown experiments in animal models. For example, a dispute has arisen whether defects of the apo C III gene or the apo A V gene are responsible for the associated hypertriglyceridaemia.[30] Association, knockout and transgenic experiments support a role for both genes; but the observation of a null allele for the apo C III gene in 140 Amish subjects and its relation to plasma triglyceride levels unequivocally establishes a role for this gene *in vivo*.[31] However, there is now evidence that a truncated form of apo A V found in rare pedigrees can also lead to raised triglycerides although one cannot study the epidemiology on such small numbers.

Some mutations are of prognostic value. Particular defects of the LDL-receptor gene can indicate whether the carrier will go on to develop a severe form of coronary atherosclerosis. Finally, methods are available to induce specific mutations in the genome so that animal models of a disease can be produced. This allows a much more thorough experimental approach than just dealing with human subjects, particularly in the use and evaluation of different therapies, although attempts to repair or replace mutant genes are proceeding more slowly.

1.4.3 Garrod's liability factors

Garrod wrote that inherited liability factors may account for the variability in the occurrence of metabolic diseases such as diabetes, gout and obesity, all specifically mentioned in his publications.[7] Such liability factors were first believed to be located at the level of enzyme regulation on metabolic pathways.[32,33] Numerous defects of regulatory enzymes were identified in various tissues of Type 2 diabetics, hyperlipidaemics and obese subjects but it was difficult to establish that they were primary inherited defects and not just secondary to the ongoing disease process. Major liability factors now appear to involve the regulation of protein synthesis by the genome and may never result in a mutant cytoplasmic protein.

Searching the genome for Garrod's liability factors for diabetes (Types 1 and 2) and atherosclerosis began in the early 1980s when DNA probes became available.[34] The search focused on single nucleotide polymorphisms (SNPs) affecting restriction endonuclease sites in candidate genes using small case-control studies or pedigrees.[35] For atherosclerosis more than 91 loci were studied around the world but none gave p-values of much less than 10^{-3}. Restriction enzyme methodology did reveal the primary genetic determinants for non-Mendelian inheritance of hypertriglyceridaemia and coronary atherosclerosis that were subsequently confirmed by genome-wide association studies (GWAS).[36,37] Many other genetic factors for non-Mendelian disorders were revealed by such studies affecting disease expression.[35] However, the search was limited to restriction endonucleases whose DNA recognition sites were mutated. The technology changed dramatically with the availability of the human genome map, the HapMap and the advent of DNA arrays (chips) that can now carry nearly 2 million DNA SNPs. This allows more complete coverage of the genome and revealed unexpected loci. The Wellcome Trust in London has used this new technology to undertake a large-scale genome-wide association analysis of seven metabolic and inflammatory diseases.[38] Cases (2000 Europids per disease) and controls (3000 Europids from two different sources) were analysed on Affymetrix gene chips carrying 500,000 SNPs.[38] To consider just the results for metabolic disease, important liability loci were observed for coronary artery disease and Type 2 diabetes. For coronary artery disease SNPs found on chromosome 9p21.3 gave p-values of 10^{-19} when compared to controls. Studies in other populations confirmed these results.[39] The variants on 9p21 do not appear to produce amino acid substitutions in cytoplasmic proteins but may produce several regulatory non-coding RNAs affecting protein synthesis. The gene for a long Antisense Noncoding RNA at the INK4 locus (ANRIL for short) is located at 9p21 and the locus appears to be a disease 'hot-spot'. ANRIL can give rise to multiple splice variants and some of these may be involved in the associations with melanoma, cranial- and abdominal-aneurysms, diabetes, gliomas, basal cell carcinoma and coronary artery disease observed at this locus;[40] however, the reasons for these associations await clarification.

More than 1,000 such loci using GWAS have now been associated with more than 150 common disorders. Many of the disorders relate to several loci having modest statistical effects but this does not mean they do not have an important biological effect, e.g. apo C III variants and coronary atherosclerosis.[31] Many loci previously found by candidate gene studies have been 'rediscovered' using GWAS, but new unexpected loci, such as ANRIL, have also come to light. So Garrod's prediction of the existence of liability factors for metabolic disease has come true almost exactly 100 years after he first stated it in 1908. We are still working on these ideas to find out how liability genes work — is it by miRNA, long non-coding (lnc) RNA, other RNA species, histone modification, DNA methylation, or some still to be discovered mechanism?[39]

1.4.4 Garrod's ideas on chemical individuality

The greatest gift a scientist can have is that of intuition, being able to guess correctly how a system works. Mendel had this to an extraordinary degree; his intuition on how monogenic traits are inherited in the garden pea kept him working for eight years in solitude obtaining the evidence to support his ideas.[41] Garrod had a similar quality of being able to guess that there must be a large degree of individual variation in metabolic pathways that partly underlies the physical differences that occur amongst people. Unknown to him an example had already been published supporting this idea. It came from Landsteiner's work on the ABO blood groups.[42] There are inherited structural variations in the mucopolysaccharides on the surface of red cells that account for the different blood groups.[43] Perhaps the most variable family of proteins is the human leucocyte antigen (HLA) system.[44] More than 2,500 variant alleles in the MHC class 1 system located on chromosome 6 produce peptides essential for normal immune function. This makes it the most genetically variable coding locus in humans (as well as other mammals). Some of these variants are useful markers for autoimmune disease e.g. the presence of HLA-B27 increases the relative risk of developing ankylosing spondylitis approximately 16-fold.[44]

Structural variation of proteins (enzymes, hormones, receptors, transporters etc.) and DNA sequences appear to be the rule rather than the exception.[46] These variants provide the genetic substrate for natural selection. Some of these variants provide a gain of function for the particular protein involved that benefits the survival of the carrier. When environmental conditions change, neutral or even deleterious variants may become beneficial for survival and reproduction and therefore contribute to the evolution of species by natural selection.[47] Garrod realised that 'such a conception [of rigid uniformity of biochemical structures] ... is at variance with any evolutionary conception of the nature and origin of species'[48] and in his Huxley Lecture of 1927 he stated: 'It is with unfavourable deviations that the student of diathesis is concerned; but if there were no beneficial ones there would be no evolutionary advance; progress could go no further ... [it is] the benign mutation which favours the individual in the struggle for existence.'[49]

1.5 Conclusion

Garrod stated his reasons for doing science: 'It is a way of searching out by observation, trial, and classification whether the phenomenon investigated be the outcome of human activities, or the more direct workings of Nature's laws. Its method admits of nothing untidy or slipshod, its keynote is accuracy and its goal is truth.'[48] He added, 'Nevertheless scientific method is not the same as the scientific spirit. The scientific spirit does not rest content with applying that which is already known, but is a restless spirit, ever pressing forward towards regions of the unknown and endeavouring to lay under contribution for the special purpose in hand, the knowledge acquired in all portions of the wide field of exact science. Lastly, it acts as a check, as well as a stimulus, sifting the value of evidence and rejecting that which is worthless, and restraining too eager flights of the imagination and too hasty conclusions.'[50]

Garrod's work revealed more about nature's laws of human inheritance than most other medical scientists cumulatively achieve in 100 years. His most important discoveries were published before World War I, when Nobel Prizes were still in their infancy. Most of the early awards were for discoveries in the fields of infection and immunity and were usually given to a single individual. A notable exception was Albrecht Kossel who was awarded the Nobel Prize in Physiology or Medicine in 1910 for identifying the four nucleic acids found in cell nuclei, a finding that eventually led to the discovery of the role of DNA in heredity. With the benefit of hindsight, one could make a good case for Garrod sharing that Nobel Prize with Kossel.

Acknowledgements

All the biographical facts, opinions and anecdotes in the text come from the only published biography of Garrod.[15] No original documents have been consulted and the author is not a practising medical historian. Grateful thanks are due to Professor G. A. A. Ferns and Professor T. M. Cox for helpful comments on the scientific parts of the text.

References

1. Garrod AE. A contribution to the study of alkaptonuria. *Med-Chir Trans* 1899; 82: 369–394.
2. Garrod AE. About alkaptonuria. *Lancet* 1901; ii: 1484–1486.
3. Garrod AE. The incidence of alkaptonuria. A study in chemical individuality. *Lancet* 1902; 160: 1616–1620.
4. Garrod AE. The Croonian lectures on inborn errors of metabolism. *Lancet* 1908; 172: 1–7.
5. Scriver CR. Garrod's Croonian lectures (1908) and the charter inborn errors of metabolism: albinism, alkaptonuria, cystinuria and pentosuria at age 100 in 2008. *J Inherit Metab Dis* 2008; 31: 580–598.
6. Bateson W, Saunders ER. Report to the *Evolution Committee of the Royal Society*, 1901; 1: 133–134.
7. Garrod AE. *Inborn Errors of Metabolism*. Oxford: Oxford University Press; 1909.
8. Correns C. Mendels Regel uber das Verhalten der Nachkommenschaft der Rassenbastarde. *Deutschen Botanischen Gesellschaft* 1900; 18: 158–168.
9. De Vries H. Sur la loi de disjunction des hybrids. *Academ Sci Paris* 1900; 130: 845–857.
10. von Tschermak E. Uber kunstlich Kresuzung bei Pisum sativum. *Zeitschrift fur das Versuchswasen in Osterreich* 1900; 3: 465–555.
11. Beadle GW, Tatum E. Genetic control of biochemical reactions in Neurospora. *Proc Natl Acad Sci USA* 1941; 27: 499–506.
12. Olby R. *The Path to the Double Helix*. Seattle: University of Washington Press; 1974.
13. Garrod AE. The Croonian lectures on inborn errors of metabolism. *Lancet* 1908; 172: 73–79, 142–148 and 214–230.
14. Garrod AE. *The Inborn Factors in Disease: An Essay*. Oxford: Clarendon Press; 1931.
15. Bearn AG. *Archibald Garrod and the Individuality of Man*. Oxford: Clarendon Press; 1993.

16. Galton DJ. Archibald Garrod 1857–1936. *J Inherit Metab Dis* 2008; 31: 561–566.

17. Meyer E. Deutsches Archiv fur *Klinische Medicin* 1901; 70: 443–548.

18. Baumann E. Zeitschrift fur *Physiologische Chemie* 1892; 16: 268–374.

19. Mendel G. Versuche uber Pflanzenhybriden. *Verhandlungen des Naturforschenden Vereines in Brunn* 1866; 4: 3–47.

20. Garrod AE, Hele TS. The uniformity of homogentisic acid excretion in alkaptonuria. *J Physiol* 1905; 33: 198–205.

21. Harris H. *Human Biochemical Genetics.* Cambridge: Cambridge University Press; 1959.

22. Haldane JBS. *Enzymes.* London: Longmans Green & Co; 1930.

23. Beadle GW. Genes and chemical reactions in neurospora. *Science* 1959; 129: 1715–1721.

24. Harris H. *Garrod's Inborn Errors of Metabolism.* Oxford: Oxford University Press; 1963.

25. Jakobs C. The Garrod Day. *J Inherit Metab Dis* 2008; 31: 557.

26. Weatherall DJ. The centenary of Garrod's Croonian lectures. *Clinical Medicine* 2008; 8: 309–311.

27. Stanbury JB, Wyngaarden JB, Fredrickson DS. (eds). *The Metabolic Basis of Inherited Disease.* New York: McGraw-Hill; 1977.

28. Scriver CR, Sly WS, Childs B, Beaudet AL, Valle D, Kinzler KW, Vogelsyein B. (eds). *The Metabolic and Molecular Basis of Inherited Disease.* New York: McGraw-Hill; 2000.

29. Gahl WA. Chemical individuality: Concept and outlook. *J Inherit Metab Dis* 2008; 31: 630–640.

30. Eichenbaum-Voline S, Olivier M, Jones EL *et al.* Linkage and association between distinct variants of the apo A1/C3/A4/A5 gene cluster and familial combined hyperlipidaemia. *Arterioscler Thromb Vasc Biol* 2004; 24: 167–174.

31. Pollin TI, Damcott CM, Shen H *et. al.* A null mutation in the human apo C3 gene confers a favourable lipid profile and apparent cardio protection. *Science* 2008; 322: 1702–1706.

32. Galton DJ. The human adipose cell: a model for errors of metabolic regulation. London: Butterworths; 1971.

33. Galton DJ, Betteridge DJ. Defects in enzyme regulation: a new approach to metabolic disorders. In: Baum H and Gergely J (eds). *Molecular*

Aspects of Medicine: Enzyme Regulation and Its Clinical Significance. Oxford: Pergamon Press; 1977: pp. 367–402.

34. Galton DJ. Molecular genetics of common metabolic disease. London: Wiley; 1985.

35. Galton DJ, Assmann G. (eds). *DNA Polymorphisms as Disease Markers.* New York: Plenum Publishing Corporation; 1990.

36. Kathiran S, Willer CJ, Peloso G *et al.* Common variants at 30 loci contribute to polygenic dyslipidaemias. *Nat Gen* 2009; 41: 56–65.

37. Schunkert H, Konig IR, Kathiresan S *et al.* Large-scale association analysis indentifies 13 new susceptibility loci for coronary artery disease. *Nat Gen* 2011; 43: 333–338.

38. Wellcome Trust Case Control Consortium. Genome wide association study of 14,000 cases of seven common diseases and 3,000 shared controls. *Nature* 2007; 447: 661–678.

39. Helgadottir A, Thorleifson G, Manofescu A *et al.* A common variant on chromosome 9p21 affects the risk of myocardial infarction. *Science* 2007; 316: 1491–1493.

40. Pasmant E, Sabbagh A, Vidaud M *et al.* ANRIL a long noncoding RNA is an unexpected hotspot in GWAS. *FASEB* 2010; 25: 444–448.

41. Galton DJ. Did Mendel falsify his data? *Quart J Med* 2012; 105: 215–216.

42. Landsteiner K. Zur Kenntnis der antifermentativen, lytschen und agglutinativen des blutserums und der lymphe. *Zbl Bakt* 1900; 27: 357–362.

43. Kabat EA. *Blood Group Substances: Their Chemistry and Immunochemistry.* New York: Academic Press; 1956.

44. Bodmer WF. The HLA system: structure and function. *J Clin Pathol* 1987; 40: 948–958.

45. van der Linden SM, Valkenburg HA, de Jongh BM *et al.* The risk of developing ankylosing spondylitis in HLA-B27 positive individuals. *Arthrit & Rheum* 1984; 27: 241–242.

46. Wolstenholme GEW, O'Connor CM. (eds). *Biochemistry of Human Genetics.* London: Churchill; 1959.

47. Mayr E. *Animal Species and Their Evolution.* Oxford: Oxford University Press; 1963.

48. Garrod AE. *The University of Utopia.* Malta: *Critiens Press,* 1918.

49. Garrod AE. The Huxley lecture on diathesis. *Brit Med J* 1927; 2: 967–969.
50. Garrod AE. The scientific spirit in medicine. Inaugural sessional address to the Abernethian Society. *St. Bartholomew's Hospital Journal* 1912; 20: 19–27.

Chapter 2

NIKOLAI ANITSCHKOW: THE BIRTH OF THE LIPID HYPOTHESIS OF ATHEROSCLEROSIS AND CORONARY HEART DISEASE

Daniel Steinberg

2.1 Introduction

Timing, they say, is all important. That is certainly true for the Nobel Prizes. If a discovery is too far ahead of itself, if it is not fully appreciated by one's contemporaries, if it therefore lies fallow for many years, then that discovery will probably go unrewarded. That was the case with Nikolai Nikolaevich Anitschkow's 1913 formulation of the hypothesis that deposition of cholesterol in the artery wall is the initiating factor in atherogenesis and coronary heart disease — the so-called lipid hypothesis.[1,2] What he showed, with his undergraduate medical student collaborator, Semen S. Chalatov, was that simply feeding rabbits pure cholesterol, and thus raising their blood cholesterol concentrations to very high levels, was sufficient to produce arterial lesions very similar to those of human atherosclerosis. No other intervention was needed — no infection, no induced inflammation, no injury, no change in blood pressure, no renal dysfunction, no diabetes — just a rise in blood cholesterol level. Nor did his rabbits smoke cigarettes! (Interested readers may want to look at an English translation of Anitschkow's 1913 paper by Pellas.[3]) Over the next two decades, a series of classic studies in Anitschkow's laboratory characterized the rabbit model in remarkable detail. His summary of that work, published in 1933, is essential reading for anyone interested in atherosclerosis research.[4] He proposed the use of his rabbit model to explore the pathogenesis of atherosclerosis, predicting that from such studies would come insights into the nature of the human disease. Sad to say, four decades passed before the importance of Anitschkow's work was fully realized and serious study of atherogenesis began. Why was his animal model rejected as irrelevant to human disease? Why was there scepticism regarding the role of hypercholesterolaemia in atherosclerosis? And why did he not get the Nobel Prize?

2.2 Were the Findings of Sufficient Importance to Merit a Nobel Prize?

Anitschkow's cholesterol-fed rabbits represented the first animal model for one of the major causes of human morbidity and mortality — coronary artery disease due to atherosclerosis. The blood cholesterol levels of his rabbits rose almost immediately and within weeks their arteries began to show raised yellow lesions rich in 'lipoids'. Anitschkow wrote:

> The blood of such animals exhibits an enormous increase in cholesterin [cholesterol] content, which in some cases amounts to several times the normal quantity. It may therefore be regarded as certain that in these experimental animals large quantities of the ingested cholesterin are absorbed, and that the accumulations of this substance in the tissues can only be interpreted as deposits of lipoids circulating in large quantities in the humors of the body.[4]

Although it was at the time largely ignored and considered irrelevant to the human disease, over the next decades Anitchkow's model ultimately became the foundation for much of modern atherosclerosis research. A major reason for the scepticism with which his work was met was that many of the attempts to repeat his work were made using either rats or dogs. These were the animals most commonly in use in laboratories of experimental physiology at the time. Feeding cholesterol to these animals did not result in the development of arterial disease: what was not appreciated was that feeding cholesterol to these animal species does not raise their blood cholesterol levels.

Anitschkow himself was aware that dogs and rats were for some reason resistant to high cholesterol intake in the diet. Presciently, he proposed that, being carnivores, they had a large capacity to handle cholesterol in the diet, converting it rapidly to bile acids for excretion. However, he also knew that rabbits were not a uniquely susceptible species. Guinea pigs and goats responded like rabbits and developed both hypercholesterolaemia and atherosclerosis.[5] Later it was shown that dogs would develop atherosclerosis on a high cholesterol diet *if* you first made them hypothyroid. The hypothyroidism caused down regulation of the LDL receptors so that the high cholesterol diet now *did* raise blood cholesterol sufficiently and now *did* induce atherosclerosis.[6]

Building the case for the importance of hypercholesterolaemia in human atherosclerosis, however, was a long uphill battle.[7] General acceptance would have to wait for over 60 years. In 1984 the National Heart Institute completed the first large-scale, randomized, double-blinded clinical trial showing that lowering blood cholesterol in hypercholesterolaemic men in the US significantly lowered their risk of myocardial infarction.[8,9] Blood cholesterol was reduced by treating the experimental group with cholestyramine, a non-absorbable ion exchange resin that binds bile acids, the products of cholesterol oxidation, and carries them out in the faeces. The resultant drain of cholesterol from the hepatocytes causes a rise in the number of low-density lipoprotein (LDL) receptors on the liver surface, a consequent increase in rate of LDL removal from the blood and a decrease in blood cholesterol. Soon thereafter the statin drugs were introduced, ushering in a new era in the prevention of atherosclerosis and coronary artery disease. The statins work in an entirely different fashion, inhibiting the biosynthesis of cholesterol in the liver, which again increases LDL receptor expression and leads to the decrease in blood cholesterol. They may also decrease hepatic output of very low-density lipoproteins (VLDL), which are the precursors of LDL. Treatment with statins can lower blood cholesterol by 30–40%[10] or by even more in high doses. Controlled clinical trials show that in subjects at high or moderate risk this is enough to reduce risk of heart attack and stroke by 20–30%.[11] Today there is no doubt that controlling blood cholesterol levels is saving hundreds of thousands of lives every year.[12] My thesis here is that the work of Anitschkow was the wellspring from which this remarkable advance in preventive medicine grew. Of course this was not evident in 1913, and the Nobel Committee can hardly be faulted for overlooking Anitschkow. There were many objections to the notion that the rabbit model might be relevant to the human disease, as discussed in more detail below. However, by 1964, when Anitschkow died, a large body of evidence had accumulated in support of his lipid hypothesis. This included the evidence that familial hypercholesterolaemia, characterized by xanthomatosis and premature coronary artery disease, was due to a single mutation,[13–15] making it almost certain that both stemmed from the hypercholesterolaemia caused by that single mutation; that coronary artery disease was more prevalent in countries with higher blood cholesterol levels;[16,17] that in any given population within a country, those individuals with higher cholesterol levels were at greater risk for coronary artery disease;[18,19] and, finally, that correction of hypercholesterolaemia by dietary intervention could reduce the risk of coronary artery disease.[20] However, the clinical intervention trials were small, not double-blinded, and not totally consistent. So, despite the considerable evidence favouring it, the lipid hypothesis remained controversial. Should the Nobel committee nevertheless have considered Anitschkow as a candidate? Did it ever?

2.3 State-of-the-Science in 1913

By 1913 it was well recognized by pathologists that degenerative changes in the arteries (atherosclerosis or arteriosclerosis, terms now used synonymously) was one of the hallmarks of ageing. However, the pathogenesis of the disease was not understood at all. Most investigators favoured the view that the lesions must be due to some form of 'injury', but the nature of that 'injury' remained undefined. In his 1933 review, Anitschkow lists more than a dozen papers describing early efforts to induce atherosclerotic lesions using mechanical or chemical injury to the artery wall (including ligation, pulling, pinching, wounding, cauterization with silver nitrate or galvanic wire).[4] He sums up the results as follows: 'these different ways of causing lesions in the arteries resulted merely in the production of inflammatory arterial changes which had no similarity with human arteriosclerosis'. He went on to note that such interventions did alter the wall of the artery in such a way as to make it more susceptible to lesion formation *if there was concomitant hypercholesterolaemia.* He cites the work of Ssolowjew who showed that injury such as cauterization could lead to 'regenerative thickening of the intima' but no lipid deposition. If, however, cholesterol feeding was started *before* the injury was produced, the site of the injury showed more severe atherosclerotic changes and greater lipid deposition.[21] Anitschkow's conclusion was that 'lesions of the arterial wall which are associated with hyperplasia of the intima create a local predisposition to the formation of lipoidal deposits, that is, to the development of atherosclerosis, *provided that they are synchronous with hypercholesterolemia*' [emphasis added].[4] This prescient conclusion has been borne out by many later studies differentiating lesions due to arterial injury without hypercholesterolaemia from those produced in the presence of hypercholesterolaemia.

2.4 Anitchkow's Contributions

Anitschkow was a keen observer and an insightful experimenter. Having established that simply feeding pure cholesterol to rabbits was sufficient to induce human-like arterial lesions (Fig. 2.1), he proceeded to explore the natural history of those lesions and the factors that influenced their development. Over the next two decades he and his colleagues established many of the key elements in the pathogenesis of atherosclerosis.[1–3,18–20] They showed that:

1) In the earliest lesions, the fatty streaks, most of the lipid was found in cells containing large numbers of vacuoles. Because lipids are extracted during the routine preparation of tissue samples, the multiple lipid droplets are seen as empty vacuoles; hence the designation 'foam cells' (Fig. 2.1).

2) In frozen sections the lipid droplets were bi-refringent. Anitschkow recognized this as representing liquid crystals of cholesterol esters.

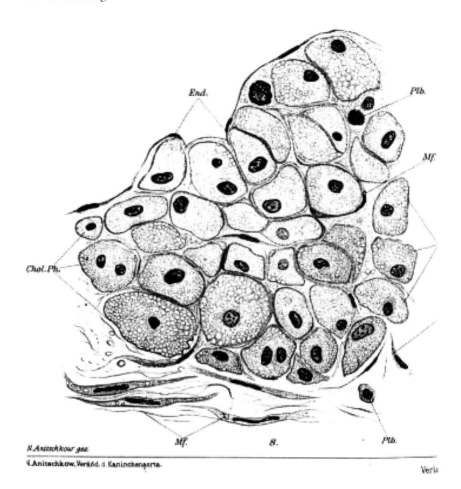

Fig. 2.1.   Anitschkow's drawing of a typical foam cell-rich rabbit lesion.[4]

3) The cholesterol-loaded foam cells were probably white blood cells that had infiltrated the artery wall. Thus he anticipated that inflammation might play a role in lesion development.

4) The monolayer of endothelial cells over the lesions appeared to be intact, indicating that the invading blood cells must penetrate between the endothelial cells. Thus, endothelial denudation, while it clearly did occur at a later time, was not a necessary antecedent to lesion formation.

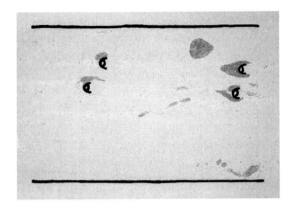

Fig. 2.2. Thoracic aorta from the same rabbit shown in Fig. 2.1. Anitschkow described the small yellowish spots of a triangular or semilunar shape, situated close below the orifices of the intercostal arteries (marked in black) and inferred that this characteristic pattern reflected the influence of hemodynamic factors determining susceptible sites.[4]

5) There was a characteristic pattern of distribution of early lesions. They were most severe at arterial branch points and Anitschkow correctly surmised that this localization was most likely determined by haemodynamic factors (Fig. 2.2). In these rabbits the very earliest lesions appeared at the root of the aorta and in the aortic arch and then proceeded caudally.

6) Over long periods of cholesterol feeding there was ultimately deposition of connective tissue (conversion of the fatty streak to the fibrous plaque) and development of a fibrous cap.

7) Early lesions were partially reversible but the reversal was a very slow process. Most, but not all, of the lipids could be mobilized from advanced lesions, leaving behind the fibrous cap and a few cholesterol crystals.

8) The extent of lesions was proportional to the degree of blood cholesterol elevation and the duration of exposure to it. Anitschkow was well aware that it was the level of *blood* cholesterol that determined the size and extent of lesions, not necessarily the amount of cholesterol ingested.

9) While blood cholesterol level is critically important, other factors can and do play a significant part. Anitschkow's dictum, 'No

atherosclerosis without cholesterol' has often been cited as evidence that he was unaware of the multifactorial nature of the disease. However, his 1933 review gives the lie to this. There he sums up as follows: 'The views here set forth concerning the etiology of atherosclerosis constitute what I have called the "combination theory" of its origin.'[4] So, it should be clear that he was fully aware that the degree of atherosclerosis, while perhaps most evidently dependent on the degree of blood cholesterol elevation, could be significantly affected by other factors such as blood pressure, toxic substances, local arterial changes and the like. In his rabbit model, however, no such additional insults or injuries were needed; hypercholesterolaemia was a *sufficient* cause. The correctness of this conclusion was most dramatically underscored by Watanabe's discovery in 1980 of a strain of rabbits that have blood cholesterol levels around 600 mg/dl and uniformly develop atherosclerosis *on a regular chow diet*.[22] These rabbits have a mutation of the LDL receptor gene identical to that found in some patients with familial hypercholesterolaemia.[23] Thus, the LDL receptor failure leads to high LDL levels which in turn initiates atherogenesis.

It is quite remarkable how well Anitschkow's description of atherogenesis has stood the test of time. While there have been, of course, many advances at the level of biochemistry, cell biology and molecular biology, the basic pathogenesis as described 100 years ago by this experimental physiologist from St. Petersburg requires little or no amendment (Fig. 2.3).

2.5 Notes on the Man and the Venue of his Discoveries

Nikolai Nikolaevich Anitschkow was born in 1885 in St. Petersburg, son of a prominent educator who served as a Vice-Minister of Education in the Russian Empire. In 1903 Anitschkow entered the Imperial Military Medical Academy in St. Petersburg. There he became a protégé of Alexander Maximow, Professor of Histology and author of what was at the time one of the most respected textbooks

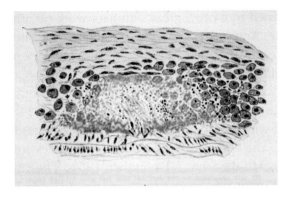

Fig. 2.3. An advanced lesion in a cholesterol-fed rabbit. Anitschkow noted the central necrotic core containing needle-like crystals of cholesterol, the foam cells surrounding the core and the fibrous cap overlying the lesion.[4]

of histology in the world. Anitschkow did his thesis research on myocardial inflammation and in the course of that work described a unique cell type that is still known today as the 'Anitschkow myocyte'. He hit pay dirt with his very first project — the demonstration that cholesterol itself could raise cholesterol levels in the blood of rabbits and induce arterial changes very similar to those seen in human atherosclerosis, as discussed above.[1,2] Shortly after graduation he went to Strasbourg to study with Hans Chiari and then to Freiburg to work with Karl A. L. Aschoff. These were the outstanding centres of experimental pathology in Europe. Both Chiari and Aschoff were much impressed by Anitschkow's work and encouraged him to continue and expand his project. Then in August 1914 war broke out and Anitschkow was called to active duty. After the war he was appointed Head of the Department of Pathological Physiology at his *alma mater*, the Military Medical Academy, a position he held until 1939. He continued to explore the pathogenesis of rabbit atherosclerosis in detail and was invited to present his findings at several international congresses during the 1920s and 1930s. So it cannot be argued that his colleagues were unaware of his findings. He intended to write a book pulling together his data and his ideas on atherogenesis and was encouraged to do so in a letter from Aschoff written in 1929: 'How is your work on your large monograph on atherosclerosis?... [Y]ou are truly destined to write a great summary work on atherosclerosis.' Unfortunately, Anitschkow never did complete the monograph but his comprehensive 52-page article in the Cowdry compendium published in 1933 tells the story well.[4]

Anitschkow was highly respected not only as a scientist but also as a capable science administrator. He headed the two Departments of Pathology at which he worked in St. Petersburg and was elected President of the Academy of Medical Sciences of the USSR (1946–1953). He died on 7 December 1964. The cause of death, ironically, was myocardial infarction.

In 1962, just two years before he died, Anitschkow established a new Laboratory of Lipid Metabolism in his Institute of Experimental Medicine and picked Dr Anatoly N. Klimov to head it. Klimov had previously worked on lipoproteins in my laboratory at the National Institutes of Health as a World Health Organization fellow. In 1966, Klimov and his colleagues reported a heroic experiment in which they had purified lipoprotein-rich serum from cholesterol-fed rabbits and transfused it into rabbits fed only chow. Because the serum lipoproteins have a relatively short half-life it was necessary to process and infuse huge amounts of donor lipoproteins to keep the level of serum cholesterol sufficiently high in the recipients. Each recipient received 14 to 25 grams of lipoprotein cholesterol intravenously over a period of 5–7 months. They developed significant arterial lesions, nicely confirming Anitschkow's hypothesis that the direct cause of atherosclerotic lesions in the cholesterol feeding experiments is simply hypercholesterolaemia. There is something satisfying about the continuity in St. Petersburg, from the first rabbit feeding experiments of 1913 to the direct demonstration of causality in 1966.

2.6 Was Anitschkow's Work Heuristic?

Not at once. As discussed above, his work certainly did not make a great splash in the early 20th century. Quite the opposite. At the time, most of his colleagues thought it was an odd result, almost certainly irrelevant to human disease. On the other hand, his findings were soon confirmed by a few laboratories using rabbits[24] and guinea pigs[25] and gradually the cholesterol-fed rabbit became a widely used model.

Anitschkow's findings were the inspiration for John Gofman and his pioneering studies on human lipoprotein fractions and their correlation with coronary artery disease.[18,19] Gofman earned a PhD in physics working with John Lawrence in Berkeley but then decided to go on to medical school. In his very first medical research venture, he took advantage of his background in physics by devising a novel way of evaluating serum lipoproteins qualitatively and quantitatively. It was based on their rate of flotation in a medium of density greater than that of the lipoproteins themselves, tracked in real time by a Schlieren optical system. In his first paper on the subject, he confirmed the findings of Anitschkow in rabbits and showed that the extent of lesions in the rabbits correlated with the plasma concentrations of lipoproteins with a density between 1.006 and 1.063, corresponding to the low-density and very low-density fractions. He and his group carried out a number of clinical studies showing that individuals with established coronary artery disease had higher plasma concentrations of these lipoproteins and that individuals with high lipoprotein concentrations were more likely to develop coronary heart disease.

Gofman's work got the attention of many scientists interested in coronary heart disease, including James A. Shannon, Director of the very recently established National Heart Institute outside Washington. Sensing the potential significance of Gofman's work, Shannon asked Christian B. Anfinsen, newly recruited from Harvard's Department of Biological Chemistry, to look into Gofman's work and to start up a new group to explore the structure and the metabolism of lipoproteins and their role in atherogenesis.

Anitschkow's findings also figured large in the thinking of Ancel Keys[16] and of William Kannel, Thomas Dawber and the rest of the group that initiated the classic Framingham studies,[26] studies that left no doubt that the chances of having a heart attack increased monotonically with blood cholesterol concentration.

In 1958, William Dock, an eminent cardiologist, reviewed 'the first fifty years' of atherosclerosis research.[27] He likened Anitschkow's discovery to the discovery of the *tubercle bacillus* by Robert Koch. In their 1998 book, *Medicine's 10 Greatest Discoveries*,[28] Meyer Friedman and Gerald Friedland include Anitschkow's discovery of the role of cholesterol in atherogenesis, side by side with Alexander Fleming's discovery of penicillin and Edward Jenner's discovery of vaccination. They make clear their admiration for his scientific contributions but include some comments on his politics. They say, without attribution or references, that 'he remained a loyal, indeed doctrinaire, member of the Communist Party and a friend of Joseph Stalin'. Referring to a photograph of Anitschkow taken in 1945 (Fig. 2.4), they say that 'One need only peruse his Slavic face, with its high forehead and cheekbones, to recognize it as the visage of a man who was neither gregarious nor benevolent. Indeed, his was the face of a full-fledged Communist of 1918 Bolshevist provenance.' The unsubstantiated statement regarding Party membership is flatly contradicted in a 2006 article by Igor E. Konstantinov, Nicolai Mejevoi, and Nikolei M. Anichkov.[29] The last co-author is a grandson of Nikolai N. Anitschkow. Noting that 'It is difficult to draw conclusions about someone's personality [from a photograph] almost a half-century after his death', they go on to aver that 'Anichkov was a descendant of Russian nobility... and never joined the Communist Party'. Why two American physicians who lived through the McCarthy era felt the issue was relevant to Anitschkow's scientific contributions is not entirely clear.

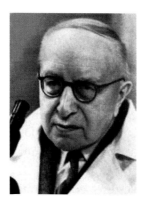

Fig. 2.4. Nikolai Nikolaevich Anitschkow (1885–1964). (Source: Khavkin and Pozhariski.[35])

Today, I think everyone in our field would accept that Anitschkow is the acknowledged grandfather of atherosclerosis research and would agree that, had the timetable been different, he would have merited a Nobel Prize.

2.7 What led Anitschkow to Feed Rabbits Cholesterol?

There is a very interesting background story to tell here. Like so many breakthroughs in science, Anitschkow's discovery was serendipitous. Many have probably assumed, incorrectly, that Anitschkow was led to do his experiment by Adolf Windaus' 1910 paper reporting that the aortas of patients with atherosclerosis contained much higher concentrations of cholesterol than did normal aortas.[30] Actually the rationale for Anitschkow's studies, as pointed out by Jeffrey Hoeg and Anatoli Klimov,[31] actually came from a 1909 paper by Vladimir Ignatowski, who was also at the Military Medical Academy in St. Petersburg.[31] Ignatowski was following up on a proposition put forward some years earlier by Nobel Prize-winning microbiologist, Ilya Metschnikow. Metschnikow had postulated that an excess of protein in the diet was potentially toxic and somehow accelerated the ageing process. Ignatowski decided to feed rabbits a protein-rich diet and look for signs of toxicity or premature ageing. He fed his rabbits large amounts of meat, eggs and milk. These diets were indeed toxic in young rabbits, affecting liver and adrenals, but in adult rabbits the major effect was the development of striking arterial lesions resembling those of human atherosclerosis.[32] Since atherosclerosis was considered one of the hallmarks of ageing, Ignatowski considered that his findings had confirmed Metschnikow's 'protein toxicity' hypothesis. One of Ignatowski's fellows, N. W. Stuckey, extended these studies and showed that the protein in the diet used by Ignatowski was actually not necessary.[33] Egg yolk alone gave the same results as did the feeding of beef brain. The lipid, not the protein, was responsible. It remained for Anitschkow and his undergraduate assistant, Chalotov, to further narrow things down.[2] They extracted cholesterol from the egg yolks and showed that feeding this pure cholesterol by itself could reproduce the vascular damage induced by the complicated diets rich in eggs, milk or meat. It was not the protein that was the culprit, but a lipid — cholesterol. From Metschnikow's point of view this would have been another instance of an ugly fact destroying a beautiful hypothesis. From Anitschkow's point of view it was the serendipitous discovery of a valuable *new* hypothesis, the lipid hypothesis of atherogenesis.

If the Nobel Awards Committee had considered Anitschkow as a nominee, would the serendipitous nature of his discovery have counted against him? Almost certainly not. As discussed by Erling Norrby in his book *Nobel Prizes and Life Sciences*, the story behind many Nobel Prizes has begun with a serendipitous or chance observation.[34] Fleming's mould-contaminated Petri dish is the best known example, but there are many others. The Prize recognizes an important discovery. It is not a prize for brilliance or for hard work or for a distinguished lifetime career. Anitschkow's rabbit experiments had not proved the hypothesis he started from — that high protein diets caused premature ageing. However, he realized that the cholesterol–atherosclerosis connection might be highly relevant in the human disease and followed the scent. Louis Pasteur observed that 'chance favours the prepared mind'. Anitschkow's mind was prepared.

2.8 Conclusion

Anitschkow was, unfortunately, too far ahead of his time. Had he died in 1994, after the statin revolution, instead of 1964, he would certainly have been a candidate for the Nobel Prize. If the policy of the Nobel Prize Committee allowed posthumous awards, then Anitschkow might very well be the nominee in 2013, the 100th anniversary of his classic paper on the rabbit model of atherosclerosis.

References

1. Anitschkow N, Chalatov S. Ueber experimentelle Choleserinsteatose und ihre Bedeutung für die Entstehung einiger pathologischer Prozesse. *Zentralbl Allg Pathol* 1913; 24: 1–9.

2. Anitschkow N. Ueber die Veranderungen der Kaninchenaorta bei experimenteller Cholesterinsteatose. *Beitr Pathol Anat* 1913; 56: 379–404.

3. Anitschkow N, Chalatow S. Classics in arteriosclerosis research: On experimental cholesterin steatosis and its significance in the origin of some pathological processes, translated by Mary Z. Pelias, 1913. *Arteriosclerosis* 1983; 3: 178–182.

4. Anitschkow N. Experimental Atherosclerosis in Animals. In: *Arteriosclerosis,* Cowdry E V(ed), New York:Macmillan; 1933: pp. 178–182.

5. Anitschkow N. Ueber die experimentelle Atherosklerose der Aorta beim Meerschwinchen. *Beitr Pathol Anat* 1922; 70: 265–281.

6. Steiner A, Kendall FE. Atherosclerosis and arteriosclerosis in dogs following ingestion of cholesterol and thiouracil. *Arch Path* 1946; 42: 433–444.

7. Steinberg D. *The Cholesterol Wars: the cholesterol skeptics vs the preponderance of evidence*. New York: Academic Press/Elsevier; 2007.

8. The Lipid Research Clinics Coronary Primary Prevention Trial results. I. Reduction in incidence of coronary heart disease. *JAMA* 1984; 251: 351–364.

9. The Lipid Research Clinics Coronary Primary Prevention Trial results. II. The relationship of reduction in incidence of coronary heart disease to cholesterol lowering. *JAMA* 1984; 251: 365–374.

10. Baigent C , Keech A, Kearney PM *et al.* Efficacy and safety of cholesterol-lowering treatment: prospective meta-analysis of data from 90,056 participants in 14 randomised trials of statins. *Lancet* 2005; 366: 1267–1278.

11. Baigent C, Blackwell L, Emberson J *et al.* Efficacy and safety of more intensive lowering of LDL cholesterol: a meta-analysis of data from 170,000 participants in 26 randomised trials. *Lancet* 2010; 376: 1670–1681.

12. Mihaylova B, Emberson J, Blackwell L *et al.* The effects of lowering LDL cholesterol with statin therapy in people at low risk of vascular disease: meta-analysis of individual data from 27 randomised trials. *Lancet* 2012; 380: 581–590.

13. Muller C. Angina pectoris in hereditary xanthomatosis. *Arch Int Med* 1939; 64: 675–700.

14. Wilkinson CF, Hand EA, Fliegelman MT. Essential familial hypercholesterolemia. *Ann Intern Med* 1948; 29: 671–686.

15. Adlersberg D, Parets AD, Boas EP. Genetics of atherosclerosis. *JAMA* 1949; 141: 246–254.

16. Keys A. Diet and the epidemiology of coronary heart disease. *J Am Med Assoc* 1957; 164: 1912–1919.

17. Robertson TL, Kato H, Rhoads GG *et al*. Epidemiologic studies of coronary heart disease and stroke in Japanese men living in Japan, Hawaii and California. Incidence of myocardial infarction and death from coronary heart disease. *Am J Cardiol* 1977; 39: 239–243.

18. Gofman JW, Lindgren F, Elliott H *et al*. The role of lipids and lipoproteins in atherosclerosis. *Science* 1950; 111: 166–171.

19. Gofman JW. Serum lipoproteins and the evaluation of atherosclerosis. *Ann N Y Acad Sci* 1956; 64: 590–595.

20. Morrison LM. Reduction of mortality rate in coronary atherosclerosis by a low cholesterol-low fat diet. *Am Heart J* 1951; 42: 538–545.

21. Ssolowjew A. Experimentelle Untersuchungen uber die Bedeutung von lokaler Schadigung fur die Lipoidablagerung in der Arterienwand. *Zeitschrift fur die gesamte experimentelle Medizin* 1929; 69: 94–104.

22. Watanabe Y. Serial inbreeding of rabbits with hereditary hyperlipidemia (WHHL-rabbit). *Atherosclerosis* 1980; 36: 261–268.

23. Kita T, Brown MS, Watanabe Y *et al*. Deficiency of low density lipoprotein receptors in liver and adrenal gland of the WHHL rabbit, an animal model of familial hypercholesterolemia. *Proc Natl Acad Sci USA*.1981; 78: 2268–2272.

24. Bailey CH. Atheroma and other lesions produced in rabbits by cholesterol feeding. *J Exp Med* 1916; 23: 69–84.

25. Bailey CH. Observations on cholesterol-fed guinea pigs. *Proc Soc Exp Biol Med* 1915; 13: 60–62.

26. Kannel WB, Dawber TR, Kagan A *et al*. Factors of risk in the development of coronary heart disease--six year follow-up experience. The Framingham Study. *Ann Intern. Med* 1961; 55: 33–50.

27. Dock W. Research in arteriosclerosis; the first fifty years. *Ann Intern. Med* 1958; 49: 699–705.

28. Friedman M, Friedman G. *Medicine's 10 Greatest Discoveries*. New Haven: Yale University Press; 1998.

29. Konstantinov IE, Mejevoi N, Anichkov NM. Nikolai N. Anichkov and his theory of atherosclerosis. *Tex Heart Inst J* 2006; 33: 417–423.

30. Windaus A. Uber den Gehalt nirmaler und atheromatoser Aorten an Cholsterin und Cholesterinestern. *Hoppe-Seyler Z Physiol Chemie* 1910; 67: 174–176.

31. Hoeg JM, Klimov AN. Cholesterol and atherosclerosis: "the new is the old rediscovered". *Am J Cardiol* 1993; 72: 1071–1072.

32. Ignatowski A. Uber die Wirkung des Tierischen Eiweisses auf die Aorta und die paerenchymatosen Organe der Kaninchen. *Virchows Arch fur path Anat* 1909; 198: 248–270.

33. Stuckey NW. Ueber die Veranderungene der Kaninchenaorta bei der Futterung mit verschiedenen Fettsorten. *Centralblatt fur Allgemeine Pathologie und Pathologische Anatomie* 1912; 23: 910–911.

34. Norrby E. *Nobel Prizes and Life Sciences.* Singapore: World Scientific; 2010.

35. Khavkin TN, Pozharski KM. Nikolai Nikolaevich Anitschkow. *Beitr Z Path* 1975; 150: 301–312.

Chapter 3

WILLEM-KAREL DICKE: THE ROLE OF GLUTEN IN COELIAC DISEASE

Chris J. J. Mulder and Karel A. Dicke

3.1 Introduction

Coeliac disease was first described in the second century by Aretaeus[1] and is now known to occur in roughly 1% of children and adults in Europe and Asia.[2] Typically it presents with symptoms and signs of intestinal malabsorption, namely diarrhoea, steatorrhoea and weight loss. In the late 1920s and early 1930s it was generally agreed that the two main principles in the treatment of coeliac disease were rest and diet. There was hardly any form of diet that had not been tried, including a carbohydrate diet (fruit, puree of potatoes or tomatoes), beef steak cure and a milk diet (2–2.5 L/day). However, as early as 1887 in the Dutch East Indies (Indonesia), Van de Burg recommended a fruit-rich diet for children with coeliac disease. These principles of dietary treatment were frequently discussed during paediatric meetings at that time. Attending one such meeting in 1932, the attention of a young Dutch paediatrician called Willem-Karel Dicke was directed to a case report presented by Dusseldorp and Stheeman describing relapses of diarrhoea that were precipitated by consumption of bread and rusks, based on the testimony of the patient concerned.[3]

From Christopher Booth's subsequent conversation with Dicke it can be concluded that long before World War II, Dicke knew that wheat products contained the offending agent: 'It was a young mother's statement that her coeliac child's rash improved if she removed bread from the diet, that alerted his interest … when he was a pediatrician in The Hague in 1936.'[4] At the end of World War II, during the 1944/1945 'Winter of Starvation', the delivery of food to Dicke's young patients in his hospital was endangered. This experience strengthened his conviction that merely eating fewer cereals and eating more other, uncommon food products such as tulip bulbs helped improve the clinical condition of his patients.

3.2 Biography: The Man who Missed the Nobel Prize in 1962

Willem-Karel Dicke was born in Dordrecht, the Netherlands, and completed his medical studies at the University of Leiden in 1929. Immediately after graduation, he joined the Juliana Pediatric Hospital in The Hague, and in 1936, at the age of 31, he became its Medical Director. J. W. Stoop, one of his disciples, wrote: 'Dicke was an outstanding clinician, scientist and manager with exceptional personal qualities. His intuition, subtle approach, analytical capacities and broad clinical knowledge made him a brilliant clinician.'[5] These qualities and his critical powers of observation led Dicke to the conclusion that wheat products contained the factor responsible for the sometimes very severe clinical symptoms of coeliac disease, at that time also called Gee-Herter's Disease.

In recognition of Dicke's outstanding clinical and scientific capacities he was appointed to the Chair of Pediatrics at the University of Utrecht and he became Medical Director of the Wilhelmina Children's Hospital in 1957 (Fig. 3.1).[6] It was to honour Dicke that the Netherlands Society for Gastroenterology instituted the Dicke medal to reward pioneering work in gastroenterology and, naturally, the first gold medal was awarded to Dicke himself.

The last years of his life were hampered by recurrent transient ischemic cerebral attacks. He sadly passed away prematurely in 1962 because of severe cerebrovascular disease. The attribution of the Nobel Prize was discussed in Stockholm by Karel Haex, Head of the Department of Gastroenterology of Leiden University, less than one week before Dicke's death. Unfortunately the Nobel Prize is not awarded posthumously.

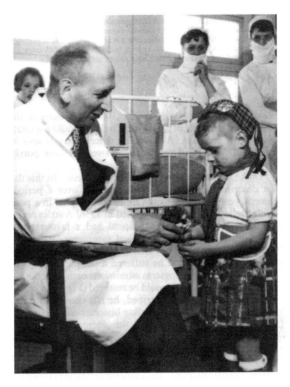

Fig. 3.1. Dicke with one of his patients at the Wilhelmina Children's Hospital, Utrecht. (Reproduced with permission of C. J. Mulder.)

Dicke had two sons, both of them doctors, one a surgeon and the other (one of the authors of this chapter) a haematologist-oncologist. It is fortunate that his widow Mrs A. Dicke-Schouten, who survived him until February 1992, was able to witness the revival of a wide international recognition of his pioneering work.[7,8] She also provided additional information concerning the development of Dicke's dietary hypothesis.

3.3 Dicke's Research into the Role of Gluten in Coeliac Disease

There are two published reports of Dicke's research on coeliac disease.[9,10] His first report about the wheat-free diet was published in

Het Nederlands Tijdschrift voor Geneeskunde in 1941: 'W.K. Dicke: A simple diet for Gee-Herter's Syndrome.'[10] Translated into English, an excerpt reads: 'In recent literature it is stated that the diet of Haas (banana diet) and Fanconi (fruit and vegetables) give the best results in the treatment of patients suffering from coeliac disease.[11,12] At present, these items are not available, therefore, I give a simple diet, which is helping these children at this time of rationing. The diet should not contain any bread or rusks. A hot meal twice a day is also well tolerated. The third meal can be sweet or sour porridge (without any wheat flour).'

The other publication is his thesis, which has been available in English since 1992.[9] His dietary studies, described therein, started in 1936 although he probably put his first patients on a wheat-free diet in 1933. The wheat-free diet had a favourable and normalizing effect on clinical symptoms, weight and growth. In his examples of descriptive cases, he has purposely chosen older children with longstanding histories of suffering, thus removing any shadow of doubt about the correct diagnosis. He excluded patients with cystic fibrosis, and faecal examinations to exclude parasitic diseases were also performed. In his thesis he presents several growth curves of children treated with a wheat-free diet. He demonstrates in long-term observations in many children that with a wheat-free diet these children gain weight and exhibit a normal growth pattern comparable with unaffected children of the same age.

After World War II, Dicke started a close collaboration with J. H. Van de Kamer, a biochemist from the Netherlands Central Institute for Nutritional Research (TNO) in Utrecht, who was the first to develop an accurate and easily available method of measuring the faecal fat-content of wet faeces.[13] Also, in collaboration with H. A. Weyers, a paediatrician from the Wilhelmina Children's Hospital in Utrecht, a method was developed which enabled faecal fat excretion in children with coeliac disease to be assessed by calculating the coefficient of fat absorption.[9,14]

Together with Van de Kamer and Weyers, Dicke undertook a controlled study in five children with coeliac disease. He challenged them with various combinations of cereal at different times and concluded the following:

1) Acute exacerbations of coeliac disease are not seen when a strict wheat-free and rye-free diet is followed.
2) The flour and not the starch component of wheat and rye is responsible for aggravating or inducing relapse of coeliac disease.
3) Flour from cereals such as corn, rice and potatoes does not provoke malabsorption of fat and therefore does not exacerbate coeliac disease.

It is quite clear from reading Dicke's thesis, as well as Van de Kamer's publication in 1952, that when Dicke went to Utrecht to perform his classical experiments he had already been convinced for many years that wheat, rye and oatmeal products were the offending agents in the causation of coeliac disease.[9,15]

The crucial experiments with standardized diets, described in Chapter 4 of his thesis, sequentially excluding or adding the wheat factor over a long period of time in children with coeliac disease, were performed on four children in the Wilhelmina Children's Hospital in Utrecht and in one child in the Juliana Children's Hospital in The Hague. The children were challenged with different cereals under an exact protocol with measurement of total faecal output, faecal fat content and the fat absorption coefficient. Based on these observations, Dicke concluded in 1950 in his thesis that wheat flour, but not well-purified wheat starch (*Amylum tritici*), and also rye flour were the cause of the anorexia, the increased faecal output and the steatorrhoea observed in these patients (Fig. 3.2).[6] The development of the gluten-free diet was based on these discoveries. Together with Van de Kamer and Weyers, he showed that the alcohol-soluble or gliadin component of the water-insoluble protein or gluten-moiety of wheat, caused the fat malabsorption in patients with coeliac disease.[16] Although these findings were rapidly confirmed by investigators from Britain, Scandinavia and Germany, doubts persisted concerning the efficacy of a wheat-free diet.[17–20] However, after the introduction of the intestinal biopsy technique for the diagnosis of coeliac disease, it became apparent that a wheat-free diet must be maintained for long periods before an adequate response occurs, as Dicke had predicted.

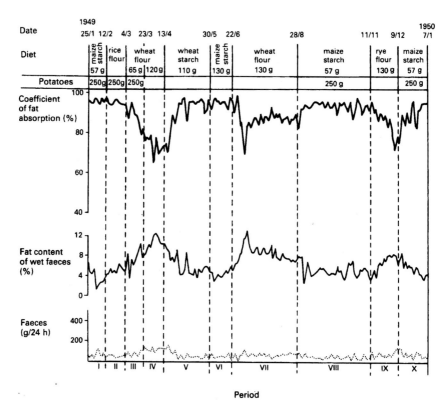

Period

Fig. 3.2. Graphical representation of effect of adding wheat and rye flour to the diet on faecal fat excretion in a patient with coeliac disease. (Reproduced from Dicke's thesis,[9] with permission of C. J. Mulder.)

3.4 Current Knowledge of the Spectrum of Gluten Related Disorders

Based on Dicke's findings, a gluten-free diet (GFD) is now recommended for all patients with coeliac disease (CD). Moreover the spectrum of gluten-related disorders in the early 1980s was simple: coeliac disease and dermatitis herpetiformis (DH) or CD of the skin. New gluten-related entities are wheat allergy, gluten-ataxia and non-coeliac gluten sensitivity (Table 3.1). The only treatment for coeliac

Table 3.1   The spectrum of gluten-related disorders

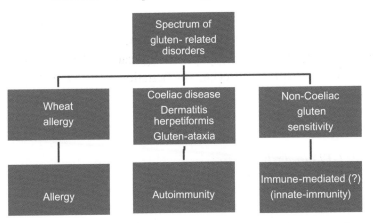

disease, dermatitis herpetiformis and gluten-ataxia is lifelong adherence to a GFD. Yet adherence by those affected is limited.

3.4.1 *Coeliac disease*

Coeliac disease is defined as a tissue-destroying enteropathy of the small bowel with clinical improvement after gluten withdrawal. The detection of CD-related antibodies in the clinical setting lowered the threshold of testing for CD. In addition, this enabled population-based screening, which revealed that CD is much more common than previously thought.[21] As opposed to CD patients identified by case-finding, most of the screening-detected patients experience little discomfort or symptoms of malabsorption. The number of CD patients that actually have been diagnosed comprises about 20% of the number expected based on screening,[22] which has not proved cost effective.[23] The consensus since the early 2000s is, in addition to case-finding, to screen only high-risk individuals (first degree relatives of CD patients and patients with Down's syndrome, Type 1 diabetes mellitus, iron deficient anaemia, transaminitis, osteoporosis and arthritis).

In symptomatic CD patients there is a clear benefit from a GFD. However, it is well known that adherence to a GFD is not only an economic burden but is also restrictive and can impair the quality of life.[24]

3.4.1.1 *Quality of life of asymptomatic CD on a GFD*

In symptomatic coeliacs a GFD induces a relief of symptoms, usually within weeks. Adherence to a GFD is accompanied in many countries by sociological, economic and psychological burdens. Symptomatic coeliacs accept this and appreciate the benefits of a GFD. Asymptomatic coeliacs will not experience direct benefits and therefore consider a GFD an unnecessary, unwanted and overdone form of treatment.

3.4.1.2 *GFD in daily practice*

GFD adherence is associated with concern over costs, availability of gluten-free products, concern with gluten exposure and the ability to follow a GFD outside the home. Some of our patients believe that they are strictly following the diet but frequently make errors due to their poor basic education and understanding of the diet.

3.4.1.3 *Evaluation of dietary compliance in coeliac disease*

Decreased compliance over time in asymptomatic adolescents compared with those who presented with typical symptoms of CD has been reported.[25] Dietary compliance is higher in families in which knowledge about CD is better and in families that belong to a coeliac association.

3.4.1.4 *Supportive treatment for those in need of a GFD*

We have to realize that the adherence to a gluten-free diet is relatively difficult. Reasons for this include:

1) Labelling legislation that allows incomplete description of food components.
2) Gluten can be found in unexpected sources, e.g. in pharmaceuticals, confectionery, desserts, flavourings, sauces or as a protein-extender in meat products.
3) In developing countries the composition of raw materials is often not exactly known, even to food manufacturers.

4) Current gluten content rules are imprecise: we advise that a gluten-free diet be as gluten-free as possible in complicated coeliacs, such as those with gluten ataxia and refractory coeliac disease. Patients and their relatives should be counselled by a trained dietician. Dietary counselling of patients and the family is the cornerstone of the treatment of CD.

In rapidly developing countries in Eastern Europe, North Africa, the Middle East, Iran and India CD has come to the attention of physicians only in the past two decades. In the past, the inhabitants of Southern India, around 500 million people, were mainly rice-eating, but now take wheat (chapattis) on a daily basis.[26] This experiment of nature provides an opportunity for research. Gluten-free foods will soon be big business but legislation for gluten labelling in these countries is insufficient, and knowledge of which products are safe is a common problem in daily life.

3.4.2 *Dermatitis herpetiformis*

This chronic skin condition is characterized by an intense burning, itchy and blistering rash. The rash is symmetrically distributed and commonly found on elbows, knees and the buttocks. Most people with DH will have varying degrees of small intestinal villous atrophy, some have none at all, but signs of enteropathy are present.

Treatment for DH is a GFD for life. In addition, in the majority of patients, Dapsone, a drug from the Sulphone family, may be prescribed to reduce the itching.

3.4.3 *Gluten ataxia*

Gluten sensitivity is a systemic illness with diverse manifestations; involvement of the cerebellum is one such extra-intestinal manifestation (gluten ataxia). Gluten ataxia is an immune-mediated disease caused by the ingestion of gluten in genetically susceptible individuals.[27] It is characterized by the insidious onset of ataxia and peripheral neuropathy. This diagnosis should be considered in the differential diagnosis of all patients with idiopathic sporadic ataxia. Early diagnosis and treatment with a gluten-free diet can improve the ataxia and prevent its progression.

3.4.4 *Wheat intolerance*

Wheat allergy is one of the most common food allergies in the United States and is one of the eight most common of all allergies. It is estimated that 5% of individuals in Westernized nations may have food allergies, although only 0.1% has a documented wheat allergy.[28] Gliadin is known as the major allergen of wheat-dependent, exercise-induced anaphylaxis ('Baker's asthma'). These patients are not allergic to other prolamin-containing grains, such as rye, barley and oats, in their diet. Hence, a wheat-free diet is less restrictive than a strict GFD.

3.4.5 *Non-coeliac gluten sensitivity*

Recent studies suggest the existence of a new condition, non-coeliac gluten sensitivity (NCGS).[29] Many individuals experience better health on a GFD, despite the absence of typical histological, serological and other signs of CD. Furthermore, most of these patients do not carry HLA-DQ2-5 or 8, which is necessary for the development of CD.

An emerging problem in our clinical practice is how to manage patients who experience gluten or so-called wheat-dependent symptoms in the absence of the main stigmata of CD.

Leading researchers in CD described 30 years ago the concept of this syndrome in a double-blind crossover trial: 'Gluten-sensitive diarrhoea without evidence of CD.'[30] Extra-intestinal symptoms dominate in our experience — fatigue, headache, lethargy, aphthous stomal lesions — and these stabilize, improve or sometimes disappear on a GFD in individuals in whom CD during a diagnostic work-up has been ruled out. NCGS patients tend to come to our out-patient clinic more frequently than CD patients and more often report severe non-specific symptoms after accidental gluten intake than do classic coeliacs. Gluten challenge, which might be part of the work-up

(30 grams daily) is in general well tolerated and accepted by coeliacs, but NCGS patients will not tolerate this for more than a few days.

Recently an Australian study provided for the first time high-quality evidence that gluten itself may trigger gut symptoms and fatigue in individuals who do not have CD.[31] Previously the perception was that gluten intolerance in individuals in Australia without CD was common but published scientific evidence was negligible.

Gluten restriction in the management of NCGS has arrived and cannot be denied any longer but we need better criteria for NCGS in our day-to-day clinical practice. The benefit is clear for the gluten-free products industry, and the economic burden on coeliacs and large NCGS groups who benefit from GFD will give rise to new products, product lines and so forth. Hopefully competition will drive down the currently high costs of a GFD.

3.4.6 *Overall conclusions*

A gluten-free diet has been the monopoly of coeliacs and DH patients since the 1950s and the spectrum of gluten-related disorders is dominated in Europe by CD and DH. Following the emergence of NCGS, especially in Australia and New Zealand, the gluten-free industry has expanded widely. NCGS may be a new paradigm that is hard for Coeliac Research Groups to absorb. NCGS does not yet explain all food intolerance but it provides a model linking a specific food component with dysfunction. For coeliacs there is a need for highly sensitive, non-invasive tests to be surrogate markers of histological recovery after GFD in order to reduce the number of endoscopies and biopsies, but current non-invasive tests are disappointing in this respect. Clinical improvement and seroconversion are no substitute for a biopsy, histological recovery being slow and unpredictable, especially in adults.

3.5 Epilogue: Willem-Karel Dicke

Willem-Karel Dicke's gift of leadership and unique capabilities enabled him to transmit to his faculty his passion for medicine and his analytical approach to resolving problems. From its introduction in 1936 until now, more than 75 years later, the number of people who have benefited from a gluten-free diet has been far beyond the dreams of Willem-Karel Dicke. His contribution to relieving the suffering of so many will have an everlasting effect on mankind, a reward of far greater magnitude than the Nobel Prize, the chance of which he missed due to his untimely death.

References

1. Paveley WF. From Aretaeus to Crosby: a history of coeliac disease. *Br Med J* 1988; 297: 1646–1649.
2. Armstrong MJ, Hegade VS, Robins G. Advances in coeliac disease. *Curr Opin Gastroenterol* 2012; 28: 104–112.
3. Stheeman HA. De intestinale infantilismus en zijn behandeling met Ventraemon. *Ned Tijdschr Geneeskd* 1932; 76: 4823–4826.
4. Booth CC. History of coeliac disease. *Br Med J* 1989; 1298: 527.
5. Stoop JW. Pioneers in pediatric medicine: Willem-Karel Dicke. *Eur J Pediatr* 1991; 150: 751.
6. Van Berge-Henegouwen GP, Mulder CJJ. Pioneer in the gluten free diet: Willem-Karel Dicke 1905–1962, over 50 years of gluten free diet. *Gut* 1993; 34: 1473–1475.
7. Pena AS. History of coeliac disease. Dicke and the origin of the gluten-free diet. In: Mearin ML, Mulder CJJ (eds), *Coeliac Disease, 40 years gluten-free*, Dordrecht: Kluwer Academic Press; 1991: pp. 3–8.
8. Van Berge-Henegouwen GP, Mulder CJJ. History of the discovery of the harmful effect of wheat products in celiac disease by Dr. Willem-Karel Dicke: 50 years of gluten-free diet. In: Sleisenger MH, Fordtran JS (eds), *Gastrointestinal Disease: Pathophysiology, Diagnosis, Management*. Philadelphia: Saunders; 1993: pp. 234–238.
9. Dicke WK. Coeliac disease. Investigation of the harmful effects of certain types of cereal on patients with coeliac disease. Thesis, University of Utrecht, 1950 (in Dutch). Second edition 1992 (in English).
10. Dicke WK. Simple dietary treatment for the syndrome of GeeHerter. *Ned Tijdschr Geneeskd* 1941; 85: 1715–1716.

11. Haas SV. Value of banana treatment in celiac disease. *Am J Dis Child* 1924; 28: 421–437.

12. Haas SV. Celiac disease, it specific treatment and cure without nutritional relapse. *JAMA* 1932; 99: 448–452.

13. Van De Kamer JH, ten Bokkel Huinink H and Weyers HA. Rapid method for the determination of fat in feces. *J Biol Chem* 1949; 177: 347–355.

14. Weyers HA. Fat absorption in normal and diseased neonates and children, especially in patients with coeliac disease. Thesis, University of Utrecht, 1950 (in Dutch).

15. Van De Kamer JH. Coeliac disease, sprue syndrome and the metabolism of fat. A review of papers by Dicke, Frazer, Van De Kamer, Tegelaers, Trap and Weyers. *Voeding* 1952; 13: 1–21.

16. Van De Kamer JH, Weyers HA, Dicke KW. Coeliac disease IV. An investigation into the injurious constituents of wheat in connection with their action on patients with coeliac disease. *Acta Paed* 1953; 42: 223–231.

17. Anderson CM, Frazer AC, French JM *et al.* Coeliac disease: gastrointestinal studies and the effects of dietary wheat flour. *Lancet* 1952; i: 836–842.

18. Soderhjelm AL. Dietbehandlingen vid coeliaki. *Nordisk Medicin* 1952; 10: 479–481.

19. Krainick HG, Debatin F. Der schiidliche Mehleffekt bei der kindlichen Celiakie. *Klin Wschr* 1953; 31: 958–959.

20. Green PA, Wollaeger EE, Scudamore HH. Non-tropical sprue. Functional efficacy of small intestine after prolonged use of gluten- free diet. *JAMA* 1959; 171: 2157–2162.

21. Biagi F, Klersy C, Balduzzi D *et al.* Are we not over-estimating the prevalence of coeliac disease in the general population? *Ann Med* 2010; 42: 557–561.

22. Collin P. Should adults be screened for celiac disease? What are the benefits and harms of screening? *Gastroenterology* 2005; 128 (Suppl 1): S104–108.

23. Mein SM, Ladabaum U. Serological testing for coeliac disease in patients with symptoms of irritable bowel syndrome: a cost-effectiveness analysis. *Aliment Pharmacol Ther* 2004; 19: 1199–1210.

24. Lee AR, Ng DL, Zivin J *et al.* Economic burden of a gluten-free diet. *J Hum Nutr Diet* 2007; 20: 423–430.
25. Fabiani E, Catassi C, Villari A *et al.* Dietary compliance in screening-detected coeliac disease adolescents. *Acta Paediatr Suppl* 1996; 412: 65–67.
26. Gupta R, Reddy DN, Makharia GK *et al.* Indian task force for celiac disease: current status. *World J Gastroenterol* 2009; 15: 6028–6033.
27. Hadjivassiliou M, Sanders DS, Woodroofe N *et al.* Gluten ataxia. *Cerebellum* 2008; 7: 494–498.
28. Inomata N. Wheat allergy. *Curr Opin Allergy Clin Immunol* 2009; 9: 238–243.
29. Sabatino A, Corazza GR. Nonceliac gluten sensitivity: sense or sensibility? *Ann Intern Med* 2012; 156: 309–311.
30. Cooper BT, Holmes GK, Ferguson R *et al.* Gluten-sensitive diarrhea without evidence of celiac disease. *Gastroenterology* 1981; 81: 192–194.
31. Biesiekierski JR, Newnham ED, Irving PM. Gluten causes gastrointestinal symptoms in subjects without celiac disease: a double-blind randomized placebo-controlled trial. *Am J Gastroenterol* 2011; 106: 508–514.

Chapter 4

RICHARD DOLL: THE LINK BETWEEN SMOKING AND LUNG CANCER

Tony Seed

4.1 Introduction

From his early years Doll was driven by one major insight — the sense that mathematical methods, particularly statistics, had a great deal to offer to clinical research. Even as a clinical student he had written a paper demonstrating the usefulness of the Chi-squared test in assessing the efficacy of a treatment, and after graduation he rapidly became involved in the famous epidemiological studies which he carried out with Austin Bradford Hill on the link between cigarette smoking and lung cancer. This work continued to the end of his life — the report of 50 years' follow-up of the cohort of GPs (general practitioners) who entered the original prospective study in 1951 was published in 2004, a year before his death. But his achievement extended far beyond this; together with his mentor and long-term collaborator Hill, and after Hill's retirement, with Richard Peto, he was instrumental in bringing epidemiology into the mainstream of clinical medicine. Furthermore, by applying it widely in the study of non-infectious diseases he helped to develop and promulgate the use of statistical methods for the objective and numerical testing of ideas and interventions in medicine. To the example and teaching of Doll and his colleagues we owe a major part of modern epidemiology and the principles of clinical trials.

Doll was not the originator of the modern clinical trial; that was Hill. But Hill was not medically qualified, and as he freely admitted he needed a clinical collaborator both to take on studies of patients and to act as an ambassador in presenting the work on smoking to a sceptical and biased audience — over 80% of men in the UK, including doctors, journalists and politicians, were cigarette smokers when the first paper was published. Doll filled this role perfectly — numerate, immensely hard-working, articulate and charming, with a slightly patrician style and impeccable clinical credentials. It was largely due to these two men that the dangers of smoking, and the responsibilities of medical and political establishments in working for its eradication, gained acceptance around the world.

4.2 Biographical Sketch

Richard Doll (Fig. 4.1, left) was born in Hampton, London, in 1912. His father was a GP, and his mother a successful classical concert pianist. He was educated at Westminster School, where he excelled in mathematics and planned initially to read maths at Cambridge; however, he failed to get an Open scholarship, being offered an Exhibition. This he rejected, and instead accepted his father's advice to study medicine. He entered St Thomas's Hospital Medical School in October 1931 and immediately became absorbed by medicine. Later, in his clinical studies during the Depression of the 1930s, his

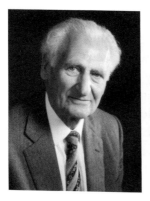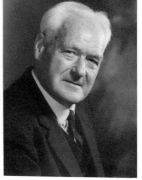

Fig. 4.1.   Richard Doll (left) and Austin Bradford Hill (right), both photographed in their 70s. (Photographs © Godfrey Argent Studio.)

experiences marked him in another way. Seeing the deprivation and malnutrition among the poor of Lambeth, and realising that much disease and premature death could be prevented by social change, he joined the Socialist Medical Association and the Communist Party of Great Britain, and campaigned actively for improved housing and health reforms. Doll never relinquished these views; in 1956, already troubled by communism's acceptance of the teaching of Lysenko, and sickened by the Russian invasion of Hungary, he left the Communist Party — and joined the Labour party.

When he graduated in 1937 he was appointed as a House Physician at St Thomas's — a real tribute to his abilities, given that St Thomas's was hardly a home to left-wing views. He went on in 1939 to pass the examination to become a Member of the Royal College of Physicians — the essential credential for an aspiring physician — and almost immediately was called up for army service. He joined the Royal Army Medical Corps (RAMC), and was drafted as medical officer to a battalion in Belgium. Less than a year later, after a tumultuous retreat lasting 10 days (his diary of which was published in the British Medical Journal in 1990), he reached Dunkirk and escaped to England. He was later posted to North Africa and then Italy, where in 1944 he developed renal tuberculosis and, on the instructions of a young RAMC officer called Paul Wood, was sent back to England. There he sought out a surgeon who he remembered with respect from his student days, and underwent a nephrectomy. He was invalided out of the army, with a 30% disability pension for life, and after a brief convalescence faced the task of finding work. He had little idea of his future beyond knowing that he wished to do research.

At this point his luck turned. He had, before the war, become friendly with Joan Faulkner, a young medical graduate who was working as an administrator in the offices of the Medical Research Council (MRC), and early in 1946 she alerted him about a research post that was being established by the MRC. This was to work for two years on a study of occupational factors in the causation of peptic ulcer at Central Middlesex Hospital in northwest London, where Francis Avery Jones had set up a dedicated gastroenterology department to study peptic ulceration. Doll applied for this post and was appointed as a research assistant.

Soon after starting he realised that his findings would have to be analysed using statistical methods, and went on a course in Medical Statistics at the London School of Hygiene and Tropical Medicine (LSHTM) run by Austin Bradford Hill (Fig. 4.1, right), who was Professor of Medical Statistics and Director of the MRC Statistical Research Unit at LSHTM, and taught the course. Hill already knew of Doll, because he was on the MRC committee overseeing his research project in Avery Jones's unit, and later he saw much of the data Doll had collected and analysed. When this study was drawing to a close in 1947, he invited Doll to assist him in a further study, which the MRC had just commissioned, to examine possible causes for the great and continuing increase in mortality from lung cancer. Doll was attracted to this; partly for the intrinsic interest of the problem and the opportunity to 'play with numbers', and partly because jobs were extremely scarce and it offered a good salary. To be presented with a compelling, important and ready-made project may also have borne some weight. Hill chose Doll because he had been impressed by his mathematical abilities and his industry; he also needed a clinician to give credibility to what might otherwise be rejected as 'just statistics'. Hill and Avery Jones, typically far-sighted, allowed Doll to continue working part-time at the Central Middlesex, and Avery Jones allocated four beds to him for continuing studies of peptic ulceration. Doll continued in this arrangement until 1969, and among other activities conducted the first randomised controlled trial in gastroenterology in the UK, on therapies for peptic ulceration.[1]

And so on 1 January 1948, aged 35, he began work with Hill and committed himself to a career in medical epidemiology. Hill was 12 years older than Doll, and already established. His teaching and publications, which included a classic textbook, had made practical statistical methods available and comprehensible to medical research workers. Hill held the Chair in Medical Statistics at a distinguished London Postgraduate Medical Institute, was (as noted above) Director of the MRC Statistical Research Unit and had (despite lacking formal qualifications in either statistics or medicine) persuaded the

MRC to carry out two randomised controlled clinical trials which successfully demonstrated the efficacy of antibiotics in the treatment of pulmonary tuberculosis.[2,3] These were the first such trials to be reported in man, and set a standard which remains today for new treatment in any disease. Thus Hill was established, influential and experienced in the medical uses of statistics, whereas Doll was a neophyte; he had published little, held no established post and if he had any reputation in medicine it was for his radical left-wing political views. In his approach to research, however, he was already a powerful force: numerate, perfectionist, scientifically rigorous and endlessly hard-working.

During the first eight years of their collaboration they published four papers (described below) which became classics and profoundly influenced the health and habits of Western society. The proportion of men who smoke cigarettes has fallen from over 82% in 1948 to 20% in 2010. Smoking is now banned in public enclosed spaces, cigarette advertising is banned almost everywhere, packets carry graphic health warnings and taxation of tobacco is relentlessly increasing. The incidence of lung cancer in the UK started to fall around 1970 and has continued to do so. The effect on the careers of Hill and Doll of this and their subsequent work was no less dramatic. Both became Fellows of the Royal College of Physicians and the Royal Society, and both were knighted. In the fullness of time Richard Doll was awarded prizes in the UK, Europe and the United States, honorary degrees by a dozen universities, the Royal Medal of the Royal Society, an OBE, the Regius Professorship in Medicine at Oxford, and in 1996 the Order of the Companion of Honour, awarded to a very limited number of citizens who have 'rendered service of national importance' — in this case to a citizen who had trouble getting a job as a young doctor because of his left-wing politics. He died, aged 92, in Oxford; his wife (Joan Faulkner, whom he married in 1949) predeceased him in 2001; they left three children. About two weeks after his death, a copy of his death certificate arrived in his own building in Oxford. He was of course a UK doctor, and so had been included in the prospective study of UK doctors' health and smoking habits which he had started with Hill all those years before.

4.3 Nature of the Medical Problem

In 1947 a conference was called by Sir Edward Mellanby, Secretary (i.e. Chief Executive) of the MRC, to discuss the increase in deaths from lung cancer which had taken place in the UK since the end of World War I, and which, based on careful data compiled by the physicians and statisticians in the Registrar-General's Office of the Government, appeared to be continuing and increasing (Fig. 4.2). The figures were alarming; incidence of lung cancer in Britain had risen by 1500% between 1922 and 1947, to a point where it was the highest in the world, causing approximately 10,000 deaths per year. Furthermore the death rate was continuing to rise by 1,000 per year.

The cause was unknown, and although there were good grounds for attributing some of the increase to better diagnosis — in particular the increased use of chest radiography and bronchoscopy — this was not accepted as a complete explanation. Various hypotheses had been proposed to explain the real part of the increase. Among the more plausible ones was atmospheric pollution, particularly from vehicle exhaust fumes, because there had been a great increase in vehicle numbers since the end of World War I. Another was an effect

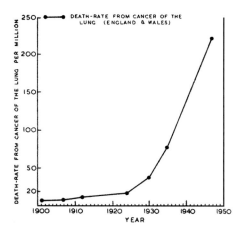

Fig. 4.2.   The problem. Death rate (per million population) from cancer of the lung in England and Wales between 1900 and 1947. (Adapted from Ref. 5, with permission.)

of particles or fumes being released from tarmac — a major road-building programme had accompanied the increase in motor vehicles. And a third was tobacco smoke, perhaps acting via arsenic, which was used in the US as an insecticide in tobacco growing and was present in trace amounts in cigarettes, or perhaps via some unknown, volatile carcinogen — though a number of animal studies with tar derived from tobacco smoke had been inconclusive and had not identified any likely agent. At that time there was no particular reason to incriminate smoking, which was widely seen as harmless, at least to adults. There had certainly been a great increase in cigarette smoking, fuelled by mass production and two world wars — many servicemen received free allocations of cigarettes and pensioners received tobacco tokens — but it was a habit indulged in, apparently harmlessly, by over 80% of men and almost 50% of women in the UK, Europe and the US.

At the MRC conference, which was attended by a small group of distinguished statisticians, pathologists and clinicians, it was agreed that there had been genuine increase in lung cancer incidence, which was unexplained. There was no consensus about the cause, which was suspected to lie in the environment. It was accepted that the matter was urgent; earlier proposals to investigate the problem had been held up by World War II. It was therefore decided that the MRC should sponsor an investigation of the problem, concentrating initially on the possible role of cigarette smoking, and Hill, who was present at the meeting, was asked to lead it. He agreed, on the basis that he would recruit Richard Doll as his assistant.

4.4 Description of the Research

The work carried out by Doll and Hill was a series of studies extending initially over eight years. Each new study was designed to test criticisms of their earlier findings, and each steadily strengthened the conclusion that cigarette smoking was causative of carcinoma of the lung. These studies have become classics of epidemiological investigation and addressed head-on the problem of 'causation rather than association' which has always been seen as a limitation on the findings of epidemiological studies.

The first study, which started in January 1948, had already been planned in outline at the MRC conference. It was to take the form of a case-control study, drawing on patients in 20 London hospitals, using a questionnaire to look for differences between patients with lung cancer, patients with other forms of cancer (stomach and colon) and a group of non-cancer patients individually selected to act as age- and sex-matched controls to the lung cancer patients. The questionnaires were to be administered by a group of medical social workers and analysed by Doll. It was to prove a *tour de force* of both administration and hard work, quite apart from its scientific value. All 20 hospitals cooperated and almost 2,500 patients, including 709 with lung cancer, were interviewed. Their questionnaires were analysed and their hospital notes examined for supplementary information; and a report had been written and presented to the Secretary of the MRC by October 1949.

Doll and Hill concluded from the study that 'smoking is a factor, and an important factor, in the production of carcinoma of the lung'. Writing about it years later,[4] Doll summarised the findings as follows:

> Our conclusion…was not, of course, based just on the finding that the relative risk in very heavy smokers was some 50 times that in lifelong non-smokers, but on the evidence that we had avoided bias, our inability to envisage any confounding factors that we could not exclude, the progressive increase in risk with the amount smoked, the reduction in risk with time since smoking had been stopped, the temporal relationships between the increase in cigarette consumption and the increase in mortality from lung cancer in Britain and many other countries, the corresponding sex differences in smoking and lung cancer mortality, and, of course, the consistency of the findings with those of the few other reported studies.

Perhaps equally eloquent was the fact that simultaneously with the writing of the report Doll himself stopped smoking. Nonetheless, when the work was published[5] the authors were cautious: 'This is not necessarily to say that smoking causes carcinoma of the lung. The association would occur if carcinoma of the lung caused people to smoke or if both attributes were end-effects of a common cause.' But they were dismissive of these possibilities on the grounds that smoking long predated the development of carcinoma, and that they could think of no possible common cause which could lead first to smoking and then to carcinoma some 20 to 50 years later.

Mellanby had retired as Secretary of the MRC by this time and been replaced by Professor (later Sir) Harold Himsworth. He was convinced by the report, but immediately saw the social and political implications and advised caution, on the basis that there might be some special effect acting on smokers in London. He recommended that confirmation of the findings be sought outside the capital. Doll and Hill accepted and apparently approved of this, and set about gathering data from chest units in other British cities, as well as in London. Within months, the inevitable happened — a very similar study, with the same results, was published in the United States by Wynder and Graham.[6] So Doll and Hill rapidly redrafted their report, without including any of the new data, and submitted it to the *British Medical Journal*.

It was published in September 1950.[5] Predictably, most reactions were hostile, and a multitude of objections were raised. Aggressive newspaper features questioned the expertise and authority of the authors; the tobacco industry questioned their data, and made much of the fact that lung cancer had arisen in a (very) few non-smokers in the study (something that Doll and Hill had expected; they never made the claim that smoking was the sole cause). Finally, professional statisticians, including the father of British scientific statistical methods Sir Ronald Fisher, and the leading American medical statistician Joseph Berkson, questioned their methods (Fisher pursued the idea that a common inherited predilection for smoking and for lung cancer explained the findings;[7] Berkson held the view that there was bias in the selection of patients[8]). Meanwhile the general public largely ignored the findings, and the *British Medical Journal*, advising doctors about what they should tell their patients, sat on the fence by pointing out that 'there is no evidence about the degree of risk which cigarette smokers take'.[9] This was true of the paper in question, but given the annual 11,000 deaths from lung cancer in Britain at the time it was something of an evasion (later studies by Peto, Doll and their colleagues[10] put the cumulative risk of lung cancer in a UK male smoker at about 1 in 6 by age 75, and similar figures have been reported in a number of other countries).

In the meantime, several other studies appeared, all supporting the original 1950 findings of both Doll and Hill and of Wynder and Graham. Doll and Hill continued collecting data from chest units and in 1952 published a second paper, merging the results with those published in the first study so that the number of lung cancer cases and controls had doubled (1,465 of each).[11] The results were almost identical to those in the first report, but in response to criticisms they had extended their analysis to look for other possible links between the environment and lung cancer: motor fumes, road dust, proximity to gas works and effects of home heating appliances. They found none. The *BMJ* was still lukewarm: 'All that these things [i.e. statistics] can do is to show that the probability of a causative connexion between an agent and a disease is so great that we are bound to take what preventive action we can.' However, this still didn't mean that doctors should advise their patients against smoking; instead it meant that the tobacco companies should seek out and remove the carcinogen in tobacco.[12]

The criticism that a statistical analysis of past events (a retrospective, or case-control study) could never prove a causal relationship had been raised endlessly following the publication of the 1950 paper, and even before the publication of the expanded version in 1952 they were planning their next innovation — a forward-looking study, which they labelled 'prospective' (today usually described as a 'cohort' study). They needed a group of subjects, smokers and non-smokers, whose health and smoking habits they could document long-term. For success, the subjects had to be a stable cohort who would take the trouble to describe their smoking habits accurately, be easy to trace and willing to respond to questionnaires regularly, and die in the UK. The idea came to Hill to use British doctors — an idea so successful that Doll later described it as a stroke of genius; over the next 50 years they were able to keep in contact with or acquire death certificates for over 30,000 doctors — 99% of those who did not emigrate. Initially they tested the idea on a sample of 200 doctors, sending a letter to the first named doctor on every fourth page of the UK Medical

Directory.* When that was successful they used the British Medical Association mailing list to send a questionnaire to all doctors on the UK Medical Register; two thirds responded, giving them a cohort of over 34,000 — it took them over a year to open all the envelopes and record the initial data. They also persuaded the Registrar-General's office to supply them prospectively with a copy of the death certificate of each doctor dying in the UK. The success of these two ideas — a long-term prospective study and a near-ideal study group — has been phenomenal; Doll himself was still publishing data on them until the year before his death in 2005.

In 1954 Doll and Hill published a preliminary report on lung cancer in British doctors,[13] and in the same year the preliminary results of a very large prospective study was published by Hammond and Horn in the US.[14] This was sponsored by the American Cancer Society, and used trained volunteers to administer questionnaires about smoking and health to almost 200,000 middle-aged men. The results of these two studies agreed closely, and supported Doll and Hill's original findings. Two years later came a second and very detailed report on the British doctors, covering over four years of observation.[15] By this time there had been 1,714 deaths in total, 82 due to lung cancer. When these deaths were analysed in relation to smoking habit, a strong relationship was shown, with the death rate rising steadily from 0.07 per thousand among non-smokers to 1.66 per thousand among heavy smokers — a 20-fold increase. The pattern held for every age group and for each year of the study, and the total mortality from cancer among smokers was in excess of that in non-smokers — in other words lung cancer caused additional deaths among smokers. Among ex-smokers, there was a steady fall in mortality with increase in time since cessation of smoking. These findings — the dose-response relationship and the reduction of risk following smoking cessation — were later substantiated further both in the US when the final follow-up figures for the study by Hammond and Horn were published[16] and in the UK when Doll and Hill pub-

---

* This sample included Sir Harold Himsworth; they could never persuade him that it happened by chance.

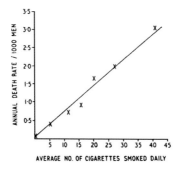

Fig. 4.3. Relationship between age-standardised death rate from lung cancer and daily numbers of cigarettes smoked by male British doctors. (Reproduced from Ref. 17, with permission.)

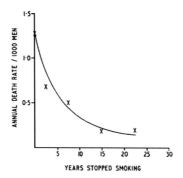

Fig. 4.4. Effect of smoking cessation on subsequent age-standardised death rate from lung cancer among male British doctors. The corresponding death rate among non-smokers was 0.07 per thousand. (Reproduced from Ref. 17, with permission.)

lished the outcomes of the British doctors' study after 10 years of follow-up in 1964[17] (Figs 4.3 and 4.4).

The 1956 paper finally turned the tide of medical opinion. Shortly after its publication, the MRC issued a report to the UK Ministry of Health (and published it in the *BMJ*[18]) that tersely summarised the evidence of a continuing rise in the death rate from lung cancer (a doubling in the last 10 years), the strong and consistent epidemiological evidence of a link between smoking and lung cancer and the absence of any evidence invalidating this link. It concluded that 'the most reasonable interpretation of this evidence is that the relationship is one of direct cause and effect'. In the same edition of the journal a leading article finally conceded, seven years after carrying Doll and Hill's first report: 'It is incumbent on doctors to do all they can to dissuade the young from acquiring a habit so deleterious to health.'[19]

There were two interesting sequels to this. First, an acid letter was written to the editor of the *BMJ*[20] pointing out that the edition of the journal which contained the MRC report also carried a full-page advertisement for cigarettes — a long-standing and profitable practice which promptly stopped. Second, the *BMJ* editorial drew a final broadside from Sir Ronald Fisher in a tetchy letter about the rejection of arguments against the smoking-cancer link:[21]

> I believe I have seen the sources of all the evidence cited. I do see a good deal of other statisticians. Many would still feel, as I did about five years ago, that a good *prima facie* case had been made for further investigation. None think that the matter is already settled. The further investigation seems, however, to have degenerated into the making of more confident exclamations, with the added avoidance of the discussion of those alternative explanations of the facts which still await exclusion.

But to all intents and purposes the battle was over. Causation of lung cancer through cigarette smoking, rather than simply association, was already strongly supported by almost all the criteria for causality that Hill himself had established[22] — the strength of the association, its consistency in numerous retrospective and cohort studies, the almost linear dose-response relationship between the death rate from lung cancer and the number of cigarettes smoked daily, and the compelling reduction in risk which followed smoking cessation; and soon afterwards the demonstration of reversible premalignant changes in the bronchial epithelium of smokers and the isolation of carcinogens from cigarette smoke confirmed the final criteria of plausibility and coherence. Doll and Hill were vindicated.

4.5 Impact of the Discoveries on Medical Science

Before the emergence of modern epidemiology, cancer, along with heart disease and stroke, was viewed as a degenerative disease, essentially associated with ageing. The work described here changed all that. It provided evidence that cancer can have specific causes, and that lifestyle and the environment might provide such causes. This chapter deals with smoking and lung cancer, and space does not allow for any wider content; but over the 50 years of the doctors' study, many causes of death other than lung cancer have been shown to have an association with cigarette smoking — coronary and peripheral vascular disease, chronic obstructive airways disease and a number of malignancies other than lung cancer are examples. Even if that were not the case, and the findings were confined to smoking and lung cancer, the statistical and epidemiological techniques which Doll and Hill developed in their studies would be monument enough. The British doctors' study was initially planned to last for five years, but it proved so successful in yielding new information that it has continued for 50 years — the most recent report, with Doll as first author, was published in 2004.[23]

In the public health arena, though, change in response to Doll's work has been very slow. The cynic, choosing to ignore how long the latency is between cigarette smoking and lung cancer, might point out that annual mortality from lung cancer in the UK continued to rise for years after Doll and Hill published their first paper in 1950 — in older men it only started to fall in about 1970 (Fig. 4.5) — and

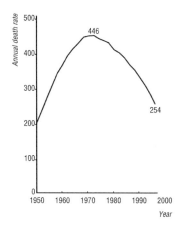

Fig. 4.5. Doll's achievement. Annual mortality per 10^5population from lung cancer in UK men aged 35–69 between 1950 and 1997. (Adapted from Ref. 10, with permission.)

remains over 20,000 now, compared to around 11,000 then. Once the death rate started to fall, however, it continued to do so and the prevalence of cigarette smoking, which in 1950 was over 80% in men, is now 20%.

Of course a political response to the risks of smoking was also slow in coming. First, tobacco was a large industry — in the 1950s, over 40,000 people were employed in cigarette manufacturing and there were 11,000 full-time tobacconists. In addition, the Inland Revenue took £600 million per annum in tax on tobacco; as the Minister of Health, Ian Macleod, wrote in a letter to a colleague when he was facing up to the need to make some public response to Doll and Hill's findings: 'We all know the Welfare State and much else depends on tobacco smoking'.[24] Second, there was inertia in central government because of the electoral dangers of intervening in a popular mass habit (in 1956, when Macleod was to make a further statement about smoking in the House of Commons, the Chancellor of the Exchequer, Harold Macmillan, noted in his diary: 'I only hope it won't stop people smoking'[25]). Initial government action was limited to a recommendation to local authorities to institute education programmes, but the pressure mounted steadily and in 1962 the Royal College of Physicians put out a widely influential report,[26] endorsing the cause and effect relationship between smoking and lung cancer and suggesting a series of measures which government could take: more public education, including information on tar and nicotine content of cigarettes; the establishment of anti-smoking clinics; more restrictions on the sale of tobacco to young people; restrictions on advertising and on smoking in public places; and increased taxation. Since then, progress has been slow, but deaths from lung cancer have continued to fall (Fig. 4.5).

In summing up Doll's achievements, some of his other interests merit mention. He left his mark in many areas of medicine: in the management of peptic ulceration,[1] side effects of the birth control pill,[27] health effects of exposure to asbestos[28] and to ionising radiation,[29] the use of aspirin[30] and other issues. And later, as Regius Professor of Medicine at Oxford, he fostered and expanded the clinical medical school there, and was pivotal in the creation of a base for medical teachers and postgraduate students of medicine — Green

College. He did this by personal fundraising on a massive scale, and academically by personal example and shrewd recruitment — a major achievement in a purist university culture which had a historical and intellectual distaste for single faculty colleges and some reservations about the academic respectability of clinical medicine.

The literature about Doll repeatedly mentions the eloquence and precision he brought to writing and speaking about his work. Here is an example,[31] wherein he is giving evidence to the House of Commons Health Committee on the scientific reasons why his original paper[5] met such a poor response:

> Three factors, at least, contributed. One was the ubiquity of the habit, which was as entrenched among male doctors and scientists as among other men and had dulled the sense that tobacco might be a major threat to health. Another was the novelty of the epidemiological techniques, which had not previously been applied to any important extent to the study of non-infectious disease. The findings were consequently undervalued as a source of scientific evidence. A third was the primacy given to Koch's postulates for determining causation. The evidence that lung cancer also occurred in non-smokers was consequently taken to show that smoking could not be the cause and the possibility that it might be a cause was inappropriately doubted.

Finally, the theme of this book demands that the issue of Doll's candidacy for a Nobel Prize be addressed. Pursuing this matter is difficult, because details of nominations and selection transactions are not revealed for 50 years by the Nobel Committee, so there is no published information about whether Doll's name was ever put forward (Bradford Hill on his own had been proposed in the early 1960s by the Faculty of Medicine at Edinburgh University,[32] but without success). We do know, however, that Doll's name was considered. In the late 1980s, the then President of the International Epidemiological Association, Walter Holland, was approached by officials of the World Health Organization for support in submitting Doll's name to the Nobel Committee. He agreed enthusiastically but on condition that Bradford Hill was also nominated; this was apparently met with incomprehension, and he heard nothing further.[33]

Feelings about this matter run high. A recent editorial in the *BMJ*[34] chronicled the work of Doll and Hill, and later Doll and Peto, on tobacco-related research over 50 years, and pointed out that the drop in lung cancer rates following this work accounted for nearly half of the fall in male cancer deaths in the last decade of the 20th century. The editorial concluded that it was 'a travesty that he never won the Nobel Prize for medicine'.

There are, however, real problems about this view, because the Nobel selection process puts great weight on the primacy of any discovery and on the contributions of individual workers. The main snag is Doll and Hill's claim to primacy of the discovery and publication of an association between cigarette smoking and lung cancer. They reported their finding internally to the MRC in late 1949 but publication was delayed (see Section 4.4) until almost a year later; during that time three papers had appeared in the US literature drawing essentially the same conclusions from similar studies — and a further one appeared in the same month as that of Doll and Hill. A further impediment might have been that, as Sections 4.2 and 4.3 above make clear, Doll's contribution to the original case-control study was that of a research assistant; the structure and detailed plan of the study was the work of Hill, and much of the support and supervision came from the MRC. Of course Doll made other major contributions to epidemiological research, teaching and academic medicine throughout his life, but it is a simple fact that the Nobel Prize is awarded for a discovery and not for a lifetime's achievement.

Acknowledgements

For biographical details in this chapter I am largely indebted to a recent and detailed biography by Conrad Keating, entitled *Smoking Kills: The Revolutionary Life of Richard Doll*, and published by Signal Books, Oxford, 2009.

References

1. Doll R, Friedlander P, Pygott F. Dietetic treatment of peptic ulcer. *Lancet* 1956; i: 5–9.

2. Medical Research Council. Streptomycin treatment of pulmonary tuberculosis. *BMJ* 1948; 2: 769–782.

3. Medical Research Council. Treatment of pulmonary tuberculosis with streptomycin and para-aminosalicylic acid. *BMJ* 1950; 2: 1074–1085.

4. Doll R. The first reports on smoking and lung cancer. In: Lock S, Reynolds LA, Tansey EM (eds), *Ashes to Ashes: The History of Smoking and Health*. Amsterdam: Rodopi; 1998: pp. 130–142.

5. Doll R, Hill AB. Smoking and carcinoma of the lung. *BMJ* 1950; 2: 739–748.

6. Wynder EL, Graham EA. Tobacco smoking as a possible etiologic factor in bronchiogenic carcinoma. *JAMA* 1950; 143: 329–336.

7. Fisher RA. Dangers of cigarette smoking. *BMJ* 1957; 2: 297–298.

8. Berkson J. The statistical study of association between smoking and lung cancer. *Proceedings of the Staff Meetings of the Mayo Clinic* 1955; 30: 319–348.

9. Leading article. *BMJ* 1950; 2: 767–768.

10. Peto R, Darby S, Deo H *et al*. Smoking, smoking cessation, and lung cancer in the UK since 1950: combination of national statistics with two case-control studies. *BMJ* 2000; 321: 323–329.

11. Doll R, Hill AB. A study of the aetiology of carcinoma of the lung. *BMJ* 1952; 2: 1271–1286.

12. Leading article. *BMJ* 1952; 2: 1299–1301.

13. Doll R, Hill AB. The mortality of doctors in relation to their smoking habits. *BMJ* 1954; 1: 1451–1455.

14. Hammond EC, Horn D. The relationship between human smoking habits and death rates: a follow-up study of 187,766 men. *JAMA* 1955; 154: 1316–1328.

15. Doll R, Hill AB. Lung cancer and other causes of death in relation to smoking. *BMJ* 1956; 2: 1071–1081.

16. Hammond EC, Horn D. Smoking and death rates — report on forty-four months of follow-up of 187,783 men. *JAMA* 1958; 166: 1159–1172 and 1294–1308.

17. Doll R, Hill AB. Mortality in relation to smoking: ten years' observations of British doctors. *BMJ* 1964; 1: 1399–1410 and 1460–1467.

18. Medical Research Council. Tobacco smoking and cancer of the lung: Statement by the Medical Research Council. *BMJ* 1957; 1: 1523–1524.

19. Leading article. *BMJ* 1957; 1: 1518–1520.

20. La Touche DMD. Cigarette advertisements. *BMJ* 1957; 2: 236.

21. Fisher RA. Dangers of cigarette smoking. *BMJ* 1957; 2: 43.

22. Hill AB. The environment and disease: association or causation? *Proc Roy Soc Med* 1965; 58: 295–300.

23. Doll R, Peto R, Boreham J, Sutherland I. Mortality in relation to smoking: 50 years' observations on male British doctors. *BMJ* 2004; 328: 1519–1528.

24. Macleod I. Letter to J Boyd-Carpenter 29 Jan 1954; National Archive, Ministry of Health, London; (NA/MH) MH 55/1011.

25. Macmillan H. *The Macmillan Diaries: The Cabinet Years, 1950–1957* (entry for 23 May 1956, p. 556). P. Catterall (ed.). London; Macmillan: 2003.

26. Royal College of Physicians of London. *Smoking and Health. Report of the Royal College of Physicians on smoking in relation to cancer of the lung and other diseases.* London: Pitman Medical; 1962.

27. Vessey MP, Doll R. Investigation of relation between use of oral contraceptives and thromboembolic disease. *BMJ* 1968; 2: 199–205.

28. Doll R. Mortality from lung cancer in asbestos workers. *British Journal of Industrial Medicine* 1955; 12: 81–86.

29. Court-Brown WM, Doll R. Leukaemia and aplastic anaemia in patients irradiated for ankylosing spondylitis. *Medical Research Council Special Report Series* No. 295; HMSO: 1957.

30. Peto R, Gray R, Collins R *et al.* Randomised trial of prophylactic daily aspirin in British male doctors. *BMJ* 1988; 296: 313–316.

31. Sir R. Doll, Tobacco: a medical history. House of Commons, session 1999–2000, Health Committee, Second Report, *The tobacco industry and the health risks of smoking*, II: Minutes of Evidence and Appendices before the Health Committee, 18 November 1999, p. 26.

32. Crofton J. Austin Bradford Hill and the Nobel Prize. In: Lock S, Reynolds LA, Tansey EM (eds), *Ashes to Ashes: The History of Smoking and Health.* Amsterdam: Rodopi; 1998: p. 213.

33. Holland WW. Personal communication, 19 March 2013.

34. Daube M, Chapman S. The legacy of the tobacco colossus Richard Doll. *BMJ* 2012; 345: 8.

Chapter 5

ALBERT SABIN: THE DEVELOPMENT OF AN ORAL POLIOVIRUS VACCINE

Derek R. Smith and Peter A. Leggat

5.1 Introduction

Communicable diseases have always represented one of the most significant threats to human health. Since the Rockefeller Foundation began the first global eradication programme in 1915,[1] much has been learned about disease treatment and prevention.[2] Arguably, one of the most successful campaigns in public health has been the development of an effective and affordable vaccine against polio. Although it first appeared in the mid-20th century, the Sabin oral vaccine continues its profound influence on public health in the new millennium. According to the World Health Organization (WHO), polio cases have decreased by over 99% since 1988, and by 2012, only parts of three countries were endemic for the disease.[3]

Sabin was a medical pioneer, helping to establish public health as a credible discipline by conducting rigorous scientific experiments and using the results to influence prevailing health care ethos. Despite his many achievements, he never won a Nobel Prize. This chapter describes the pioneering contributions of Albert Sabin and how his vaccine had a profound impact on the global rate of polio infections. Since many different factors influenced health care during the last century, we describe his involvement with respect to prevailing scientific paradigms and public health issues of the time. Our chapter also outlines the basic epidemiology of poliovirus and the historical development of an effective vaccine, both by Sabin and by others.

5.2 The Early Years of Albert Sabin

Albert Bruce Sabin was born on 26 August 1906 in Bialystok, Russian Empire, in what is now Poland.[4] In 1921, the Sabin family emigrated to the United States to avoid increasing persecution of Jewish citizens in what was then Imperial Russia.[5] Suspecting his future lay in academic pursuits, Sabin entered and later graduated from New York University (NYU) in 1928. He subsequently enrolled in medical school at the same institute, and his early interest in experimentation yielded a new method for the rapid typing of pneumococci.[4] With financial aid from various fellowships and scholarships, he graduated with a medical degree from NYU in 1931, which was also the year New York experienced a large polio epidemic. This event no doubt influenced the young graduate and helped sow the seed for his lifelong interest in medical research.[5]

After graduating from NYU, Sabin worked as a House Physician at Bellevue Hospital in New York, between 1932 and 1933. In 1934 he moved to the Lister Institute of Preventive Medicine in London to take up a position as a National Research Council Fellow.[4] Sabin returned to New York a year later, and subsequently joined the Rockefeller Institute for Medical Research. After four years in New York, he moved to the University of Cincinnati Children's Hospital and created a research laboratory which would later develop his landmark vaccine. Sabin served in the US Army Medical Corps during World War II as a Lieutenant Colonel, during which time he studied various diseases that affected American troops stationed abroad.[4] Based on this experience, Sabin developed experimental vaccines against Dengue fever for troops in the South Pacific theatre of war and a vaccine against Japanese encephalitis virus. As a result, his Japanese encephalitis vaccine was administered to around 70,000 soldiers who were, at the time, preparing to invade Japan.[4] Following the cessation of hostilities at the end of the war, Sabin continued his research on polio vaccines. This coincided with an interesting historical phase for public health, as a large proportion of the international scientific effort which had previously focused on war-related activities was now free to focus on peacetime pursuits.

5.3 The Historical Development of Poliovirus Knowledge

Sporadic polio cases have probably affected humans since time immemorial, with atrophied limbs among young people being depicted in ancient Egypt.[6] The first complete clinical description of the disease occurred in 1840, after which time reports gradually began to become more frequent, more severe and more widespread.[7] Even so, the epidemiology of polio took some time to be completely understood. By the early 20th century, it was well known that epidemics usually radiated from a central point; however polio's pattern of spread appeared erratic as many infected people had no history of contact with a known source.[8] Part of the problem was early confusion regarding the biological infection route. In 1908 for example, it was thought that poliovirus entered the human body via inhalation,[9] a hypothesis which had arisen via the demonstration of nasal lesions in some infected cases. Consequently, initial polio research focused on the experimental transmission of disease to monkeys.[8]

Albert Sabin was already working in this field by the 1930s, and in 1931 published his first article on polio.[10] This was an important step as the possibility of an oral-alimentary infection route for polio was now being seriously considered by scientific researchers. Furthermore, during 1932, high levels of the virus were demonstrated in the faeces of polio patients and healthy carriers.[8] The concept of alternative sites for transmission also began to simultaneously falter when a 1936 publication showed that nasal lesions existed only in experimental monkeys who had contracted polio via a respiratory route.[9] Other animal models were also being developed for polio experimentation, with poliovirus first being grown experimentally in mice in 1939.[8] In 1940, the Yale Poliomyelitis Study Unit began testing for poliovirus among New York sewage and found it to be highly prevalent. Sewage testing not only showed that the virus was excreted from carriers in this manner but that a large number of infected persons were probably asymptomatic. Melnick and colleagues later suggested a ratio of about 100 sub-clinical infections for every paralytic case.[8] By the 1950s, it had been established that poliovirus could be isolated from several species of flies during summer epidemics. However, flies emerging from maggots that had been experimentally fed poliovirus were shown to be free from the agent;[11] a finding which cast doubt on flies as a significant reservoir.

Research on poliovirus immunology was also developing during this period, and by 1952 it had been established that neutralizing antibodies for poliovirus were demonstrable in patients at or shortly after the onset of symptoms, and increasingly so during convalescence.[12,13] Experimental studies on poliomyelitis variants were also continuing in the Sabin laboratory.[14] As the 20th century progressed, the propensity for polio to appear in community outbreaks firmly entrenched it as an important issue for public health researchers. Furthermore, the implication of human sewage as a possible vector suggested that public health interventions would need to be incorporated into any type of control programme. Although some early 20th century experts had tried to define polio simply as a disease of the poor and unclean,[15] large concentrations of the virus in sewage helped foster a new understanding that it was a disease that could be contracted by anyone, given the appropriate exposure.

5.4 The Development of a Poliovirus Vaccine

During many of the experiments mentioned earlier, and for a variety of reasons, it had become apparent to Sabin that oral exposure might be a promising direction from which to develop a vaccine. Chief among them was the fact that although polio was seemingly endemic in developing countries, not everyone suffered a paralytic attack. Similarly, the high titres found in first-world sewage indicated that gastric ingestion may not always result in paralysis. Sabin must have been considerably encouraged in 1952 when a large field trial demonstrated that passive antibodies offered a short-term protective effect against paralytic polio.[8]

At this point it is important to note that Albert Sabin was not the only person, nor the first, to make groundbreaking discoveries in polio research. Karl Landsteiner, for example, had demonstrated the viral origins of polio by transmitting the disease from infected humans to monkeys in 1908. He would later go on to discover human blood groups, for which he received the Nobel Prize in 1930.[6] The first human administration of an experimental oral polio vaccine was undertaken by Koprowski and colleagues in February 1950, after which time a further 19 children were orally vaccinated and all developed antibodies.[16] In 1955, an inactivated polio vaccine (administered by intramuscular injection) was developed by Jonas Salk and rapidly adopted throughout the US.[17] Although an immediate decline in cases was noted, the trend levelled off and then reversed by 1959, despite the administration of approximately 300 million doses.[18] There were several reasons for this, chief among them being that circulating antibody titres seemed to decline significantly within a few years of vaccination. Secondly, polio had not been totally eradicated and wild types of the virus continued to circulate, causing localized outbreaks in partly immunized or non-immunized individuals. Tragically, in a highly publicized incident in 1955, over 260 people contracted polio from the vaccine and 11 died.[17] It was later learned that poliovirus could still grow within the gut of vaccinated persons, before being transmitted to the non-immunized.[7] Another disadvantage of the Salk vaccine was that around 1,500 monkeys were needed to produce one million inactivated doses.[18] As monkeys represented a critical step in the process, this large demand from a single branch of medical science began to lead to a shortage of animals.

Throughout this time, Sabin maintained that intensive widespread vaccination with a live vaccine (as opposed to Salk's inactivated 'dead' vaccine) could interrupt disease transmission at lower overall levels of vaccination coverage than ongoing or routine programmes.[19] An oral vaccine could also be more easily administered and better tolerated as a mass public health measure. Furthermore, live oral viruses would be effective at imitating natural infection as they could establish an asymptomatic infection within the gut, which would in turn stimulate immune response and the excretion of local and systematic antibodies. Building on these theories, Sabin developed an oral vaccine consisting of three attenuated strains (one from each serotype) of live poliovirus.[20]

5.5 Albert Sabin: Publications and Recognition

On 6 August 1960, Albert Sabin published his landmark article entitled 'Live, Orally Given Poliovirus Vaccine' in the prestigious *Journal of the American Medical Association* (*JAMA*).[21] In this manuscript, Sabin described the results of a large study where the newly developed trivalent oral vaccine was administered over a period of four days to over 26,000 children, representing 86% of all those aged below 11 years. Due to the self-limiting nature of poliovirus, a second dosing was needed to achieve almost complete immunization coverage. This point was confirmed with increased understanding of poliovirus epidemiology in later years, when it was shown that transmission can be effectively interrupted by achieving high population immunity.[2] So important was Sabin's article to medical science that it was republished by *JAMA* in 1984,[22] and later by the WHO in 1999.[23]

In 1961, monovalent strains for the Sabin vaccine were licensed in the US, with a trivalent vaccine following soon after. In 1962, the world's first nationwide polio vaccination campaign was undertaken in Cuba,[24] and its early successes helped lay the foundation for a worldwide polio eradication strategy.[25] The significant contribution to polio vaccine by the USSR is also worth noting, as it followed a fortuitous meeting in 1956 between Albert Sabin and Mikhail Chumakov.[26] During this meeting, Sabin provided experimental results, and more importantly his strains of polio vaccine to Chumakov, who subsequently began to produce it for use in his homeland. At that time, polio was a widespread public health issue throughout the USSR, a fact which enabled Chumakov to undertake trials of the vaccine, first in Estonia and later in Lithuania. By 1959, over 15 million Soviets, mainly children, had been inoculated with the Sabin vaccine.[26]

The Russian success story constituted a large body of evidence which was deliberated upon by the Division of Biological Standards of the US National Institutes of Health, who eventually recommended all three strains of the Sabin vaccine for licensing. Between 1962 and 1964, around 100 million Americans of all ages received the new Sabin oral vaccine. Large, public health field trials were also conducted in Czechoslovakia, but it was the widespread use in Brazil in 1980 which demonstrated that polio eradication might be feasible on a worldwide scale. These successes prompted the World Health Assembly (a decision-making body of the WHO) in 1988 to adopt a goal of global polio eradication.[27] Although their initial goal has not yet been reached, numerous public health achievements have nevertheless been made with respect to polio. By 1995 for example, around 80% of all children worldwide had received the three required doses of vaccine in the first year of life, and this was preventing at least 400,000 polio cases annually.[7]

5.6 Why the Sabin Vaccine was a Pioneering Development

Albert Sabin was not the first person to consider the eradication of a human pathogen, as major disease eradication schemes were being undertaken by medical researchers throughout the last century. Nevertheless, there were a few good reasons why Sabin's oral vaccine was a pioneering step, and why he was able to make such a significant contribution to public health. Firstly, there was the issue of demand. Although polio may be transmitted by various animals (such as flies) in certain situations,[11] humans represent the only known reservoir.[7] The disease spreads rapidly through infected households and is often present in urban sewage, being most likely spread from infectious faeces by contaminated fingers. When Sabin was young, large polio epidemics were spreading across the US and Europe. In the summer of 1916 for example, the US experienced 27,000 cases of paralytic polio and 6,000 related deaths.[7] These outbreaks caused anxiety, horror and political unrest in the general population.[6] People fleeing New York during the polio epidemic of 1931, for example, were actually turned back at gunpoint by some residents of neighbouring towns, such was their fear of the disease. This was despite the fact that it killed fewer children than other epidemics of the day, including diphtheria, whooping cough or measles.[15] As a result of this widespread public concern, the need for an effective vaccine became paramount in the eyes of not only public health experts, but also the general public and those who governed them.

Secondly, there was Sabin's continual insistence that a live oral vaccine was superior to an inactivated one. Indeed, Sabin once stated that his mission was to 'kill the killed [Salk] vaccine'.[4] This was a shrewd scientific decision given the prevailing scientific paradigms of the day. An oral vaccine was easier to administer, and it provided longer lasting immunity from fewer doses. Importantly, an oral vaccine would also help stimulate local and systemic immunity, which would in turn help prevent its spread from asymptomatic people. Nonetheless, Sabin probably benefited from a certain amount of luck when choosing his live strains. In 1950 for example, Koprowski and Cox began experiments with a slightly different, rodent-adapted Type 2 strain, which was subsequently fed to millions throughout the world. Unfortunately, the father of a child receiving Cox vaccination developed paralysis and died.[7] When properties of the Cox virus were recovered from his brain tissue, the strain was withdrawn, paving the way for the widespread adoption of the (alternative) Sabin trivalent oral vaccine.

5.7 The Sabin Vaccine Today

Over two decades after his death, the Sabin oral vaccine continues to exert its profound influence on public health the world over. By the year 2000, it had been estimated that 350,000 lives were being saved each year by the oral vaccine, with an annual global saving of 1.5 billion US dollars.[2] According to the World Health Organization (WHO), polio cases have decreased over 99% since 1988, and by 2012 only parts of three countries worldwide were still endemic for the disease.[3] Despite these enormous savings in lives and dollars, and the associated money-making potential, it seems that Albert Sabin's motivation was not financial, having donated his carefully devised strains of poliovirus to the WHO in 1972. This unprecedented humanitarian gesture was intended to increase the availability of an effective vaccine for developing countries, and was remarkably successful from both a scientific and humanitarian point of view.[28] Research continues on the Sabin vaccine, including a renewed interest in new and novel uses for it.[29–31] Since 1993, the Sabin Vaccine

Institute has continued his work and now focuses on vaccine development, delivery and distribution for other diseases such as rubella, rotavirus and hookworm, as well as polio.[32]

5.8 Albert Sabin, Polio and the Nobel Prize

The Nobel Prize was founded following the death of Alfred Nobel in 1896, who had stipulated that his fortune be used for prizes awarded annually in the fields of chemistry, physics, physiology or medicine, literature and peace.[33] The procedures for selection of award recipients have evolved over the past century, as Nobel's final Will only offered limited guidance on how the selection process should actually work.[34] However, it is important to note that he did provide some important distinctions for when the Nobel Prize was awarded in the field of physiology or medicine — that the main emphasis should be scientific originality and that it be given exclusively for a 'discovery'.[34] When considering the global eradication of polio therefore, it is reasonable to assume that Nobel himself might have considered the development of an inactivated or live vaccine worthy of the prize that bears his name.[35] If so, it is interesting to consider why a Nobel Prize was not awarded to Albert Sabin or any other pioneering polio vaccine researchers such as Salk, Younger, Koprowski or Cox. Although much of this debate and story behind it has been examined by Erling Norrby in his book, *Nobel Prizes and Life Sciences*,[6] it is worth recounting some of the main points here.

Perhaps one of the more contentious aspects in this debate occurred in 1954 when John F. Enders, Thomas H. Weller and Frederick C. Robbins received the Nobel Prize in Physiology or Medicine for their discovery of polio viruses' ability to grow in various types of non-nervous tissue. Their story actually begins a few years earlier, in 1940, when Enders first engaged Weller (a medical student at the time) for a research project, after which they were also joined by Robbins (a medical school classmate). Through a series of experiments conducted in 1948, the trio was able to demonstrate that poliovirus did not necessarily need nervous tissue for its growth — a pioneering step that helped overcome the widely held perception that viral replication was only possible in the nervous system. Aside from this breakthrough and its implication for polio, their discovery was also significant in furthering the understanding of other medically important viruses.[36] As a result, Enders (alone) was first nominated for a Nobel Prize in 1952, and again in 1953. Enders received a further nine nominations in 1954, two of which now included Weller and Robbins.

Interestingly, in the same year, the Nobel Committee had originally proposed that Vincent du Vigneaud be awarded the Nobel Prize in Physiology or Medicine for his discovery of the structure of vasopressin and oxytocin.[36] But by September 1954, the committee had instead recommended that Enders, Robbins and Weller be jointly awarded it for their discovery of the capacity of poliovirus to grow in different tissue cultures from primates.[35] In the following year, 1955, Jonas Salk was first nominated for the Nobel Prize in Physiology or Medicine, followed by joint nominations for Hilary Koprowski and Albert Sabin in 1958. But it was not to be — none of them were ever selected by the Nobel Committee.

Although Albert Sabin never received the Nobel Prize, he still received numerous accolades for his work with the oral polio vaccine, including over 40 honorary degrees, the US National Medal of Science, the Presidential Medal of Freedom, the Medal of Liberty, the Order of Friendship Among Peoples (Russia), the Ordem Cruzeiro do Sul Grande Oficial and the Gran Cruz da Ordem do Rio Branco (Brazil),[37] and the Lasker Clinical Research Award in 1965 (Fig. 5.1). By all accounts, Albert Sabin was a stubborn but eloquent speaker, and therefore difficult to defeat in scientific arguments. When asked about his prime competitor Jonas Salk, Sabin once declared that the Salk vaccine was 'pure kitchen chemistry'.[4] Sabin was not alone in this criticism, as many in the scientific community also felt that Salk had not really discovered anything new, rather he had simply produced a polio vaccine from techniques founded by others.[17]

5.9 Epilogue

Albert Sabin entered a world where the average lifespan of males was 47 years, and for females it was 51 years. Tuberculosis, pneumonia

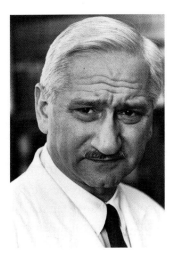

Fig. 5.1. Albert Sabin, 1906–1993. (Courtesy of the Albert and Mary Lasker Foundation.)

and heart disease were the biggest killers, diseases for which adequate preventive measures were largely unavailable. Theories of disease causation were slowly being refined following the groundbreaking work of Pasteur and others, but a complete transition to the modern understanding of disease causation had not yet been achieved. By the time of Sabin's graduation from university in 1931, the average human lifespan had risen to 60 years for men and 63 years for women. In the 29-year gap between the publication of Sabin's first paper in 1931[10] and his landmark *JAMA* article in 1960,[21] worldwide infant mortality had been reduced more than three-fold and average lifespan had also increased by almost 150% in women. By the time of his death in 1993, male and female life expectancy had increased to 72 and 79 years, respectively.[38]

Albert Sabin retired from full-time work in 1986 at the age of 80, although he continued publishing[39] right up until his death from heart failure in March 1993.[40] He was buried in Arlington National Cemetery, an honour reserved for those who served in the US military. Over the course of his life, spectacular achievements in public health (including the polio vaccine) had reduced infant mortality ten-fold. Infectious disease had all but disappeared as the prime cause of mortality within industrialized countries. His early hypotheses on the theory and causations of large-scale public health epidemics would later be shown to be fundamentally correct.[41] On the other hand, it has been suggested that Sabin's effectiveness was often compromised by his stubbornness, an inadequate concern for the interests of certain stakeholders and a general inability to acknowledge the shortcomings of the oral polio vaccine.[42] It is worth noting, however, that both the inactivated (Salk) and live (Sabin) vaccines are still used today, and both have their share of advantages and disadvantages.[43] Although Sabin was not alone in his desire to eradicate diseases, his achievements remain profound and far-reaching for public health, even when considering the continual advance of medical technology after his death. That he never won a Nobel Prize is probably irrelevant nowadays, as Sabin's work has clearly cemented his place as one of history's great medical pioneers.

Acknowledgements

This chapter represents a revised and expanded version of a previously published article:

Smith DR, and Leggat PA. Pioneering figures in medicine. Albert Bruce Sabin — Inventor of the oral polio vaccine. *Kurume Medical Journal* 2005; 52: 111–116 (available online at: https://www.jstage.jst.go.jp/article/kurumemedj/52/3/52_3_111/_article).

References

1. Miller M, Barrett S, Henderson DA. Control and Eradication. In: Jamison DT, Breman JG, Measham AR (eds), *Disease Control Priorities in Developing Countries.* 2nd Edition. Washington: World Bank; 2006: pp. 1163–1176.

2. Aylward B, Hennessey KA, Zagaria N, Olive JM, Cochi S. When is a disease eradicable? 100 years of lessons learned. *Am J Public Health* 2000; 90: 1515–1520.

3. *World Health Organization (WHO) Media Centre Webpage. Poliomyelitis, Factsheet No. 114.* Available online at: http://www.who.int/mediacentre/factsheets/fs114/en/ (Accessed: 16 December 2012).
4. Melnick JL, Horaud F. Albert B. Sabin. *Biologicals* 1993; 21: 297–303.
5. MacLaughlin S. Dr. Albert Sabin. *Prim Care Update Ob Gyns* 2003; 10: 129–130.
6. Norrby E. *Nobel Prizes and Life Sciences.* Singapore: World Scientific Publishing; 2010.
7. Melnick JL. Current status of poliovirus infections. *Clinical Microbiology Reviews* 1996; 9: 293–300.
8. Melnick JL. The discovery of the enteroviruses and the classification of poliovirus among them. *Biologicals* 1993; 21: 305–309.
9. Horaud F. Albert B. Sabin and the development of oral poliovaccine. *Biologicals* 1993; 21: 311–316.
10. Sabin AB. Purification of poliomyelitis virus by adsorption and elution. *Proc Soc Exp Biol Med* 1931; 29: 59–62.
11. Melnick JL, Penner LR. The survival of poliomyelitis and Coxsackie viruses following their ingestion by flies. *J Exp Med* 1952; 96: 255–271.
12. Sabin AB. Transitory appearance of type 2 neutralizing antibody in patients infected with type 1 poliomyelitis virus. *J Exp Med* 1952; 96: 99–106.
13. Winsser J, Sabin AB. Levels of homotypic neutralizing antibody in human poliomyelitis three years after infection. *J Exp Med* 1952; 96: 477–490.
14. Sabin AB, Hennessen WA, Winsser J. Studies on variants of poliomyelitis virus. I. Experimental segregation and properties of avirulent variants of three immunologic types. *J Exp Med* 1954; 99: 551–576.
15. Baker JP. Immunization and the American way: 4 childhood vaccines. *American Journal of Public Health* 2000; 90: 199–207.
16. Koprowski H. First decade (1950–1960) of studies and trials with the polio vaccine. *Biologicals* 2006; 34: 81–86.
17. Kleiss KM. Dr. Jonas Salk. *Prim Care Update Ob Gyns* 2003; 10: 127–128.
18. Hinman AR. Landmark perspective: Mass vaccination against polio. *JAMA* 1984; 251: 2994–2996.

19. de Quadros CA, Henderson DA. Disease eradication and control in the Americas. *Biologicals* 1993; 21: 335–343.

20. Minor PD, Macadam AJ, Stone DM *et al.* Genetic basis of attenuation of the Sabin oral poliovirus vaccines. *Biologicals* 1993; 21: 357–363.

21. Sabin AB, Ramos-Alvarez M, Alvarez-Amezquita J *et al.* Live, orally given poliovirus vaccine. Effects of rapid mass immunization on population under conditions of massive enteric infection with other viruses. *JAMA* 1960; 173: 1521–1526.

22. Sabin AB, Ramos-Alvarez M, Alvarez-Amezquita J *et al.* Landmark article Aug 6, 1960: Live, orally given poliovirus vaccine. Effects of rapid mass immunization on population under conditions of massive enteric infection with other viruses. By Albert B. Sabin, Manuel Ramos-Alvarez, Jose Alvarez-Amezquita, William Pelon, Richard H. Michaels, Ilya Spigland, Meinrad A. Koch, Joan M. Barnes, and Johng S. Rhim. *JAMA* 1984; 251: 2988–2993.

23. Sabin AB, Ramos-Alvarez M, Alvarez-Amezquita J *et al.* Live, orally given poliovirus vaccine. Effects of rapid mass immunization on population under conditions of massive enteric infection with other viruses. 1960. *Bull World Health Organ* 1999; 77: 196–201.

24. Cruz RR. Cuba: Mass Polio Vaccination Program, 1962–1982. *Reviews of Infectious Diseases* 1984; 6: S408–S412.

25. Lago PM. Eradication of poliomyelitis in Cuba: A historical perspective. *BullWorld Health Organ* 1999; 77: 681–687.

26. Agol VI, Drozdov SG. Russian contribution to OPV. *Biologicals* 1993; 21: 321–325.

27. Ward NA, Milstien JB, Hull HF *et al.* The WHO-EPI initiative for the global eradication of poliomyelitis. *Biologicals.* 1993; 21: 327–333.

28. Magrath D, Reeve P. On the role of the World Health Organization in the development of Sabin vaccines. *Biologicals* 1993; 21: 345–348.

29. Racaniello VR. Infectious cDNA, cell receptors and transgenic mice in the study of Sabin's poliovirus vaccines. *Biologicals* 1993; 21: 365–369.

30. Wimmer E, Nomoto A. Molecular biology and cell-free synthesis of poliovirus. *Biologicals* 1993; 21: 349–356.

31. Girard M, Martin A, van der Werf S. Potential use of poliovirus as a vector. *Biologicals* 1993; 21: 371–377.

32. *Sabin Vaccine Institute Website.* Available online at: http://www.sabin. org/ (Accessed: 13 November 2012).
33. Thompson G. Preface. In: Thompson, G (ed.), *Nobel Prizes that Changed Medicine.* London: Imperial College Press; 2012: pp. ix–xii.
34. Norrby E. Unusual Nobel Prizes in Physiology or Medicine. In: Norrby, E, *Nobel Prizes and Life Sciences.* Singapore: World Scientific Publishing; 2010: pp. 144–150.
35. Norrby E, Prusiner SB. Polio and Nobel prizes: Looking back 50 years. *Ann Neurol* 2007; 61: 385–395.
36. Norrby E. Polio and Nobel Prizes. In: Norrby, E, *Nobel Prizes and Life Sciences.* Singapore: World Scientific Publishing; 2010: pp. 124–143.
37. *Sabin Vaccine Institute Webpage. The Legacy of Albert B. Sabin.* Available online at: http://www.sabin.org/legacy-albert-b-sabin (Accessed: 8 February 2013).
38. *UC Berkeley Website, Department of Demography.* Available online at: http://demog.berkeley.edu/~andrew/1918/figure2.html (Accessed: 5 February 2013).
39. Sabin AB. Reflections on the qualitative and quantitative aspects of neurovirulence of different polioviruses. *Dev Biol Stand* 1993; 78: 3–7.
40. Grouse LD. Albert Bruce Sabin. *JAMA* 1993; 269: 2140.
41. Dowdle WR. The principles of disease elimination and eradication. *Bull World Health Organ* 1998; 76 Suppl 2: 22–25.
42. Hampton L. Albert Sabin and the Coalition to Eliminate Polio from the Americas. *Am J Public Health* 2009; 99: 34–44.
43. Shibuya K, Murray CJL. Poliomyelitis. In: Murray CJL, Lopez AD, Mathers CD (eds), *The Global Epidemiology of Infectious Diseases.* Geneva: World Health Organization; 2004: pp. 111–149.

Chapter 6

RENÉ FAVALORO: PIONEER OF CORONARY ARTERY SURGERY

Stephen Westaby

6.1 The Beginning

René Geronimo Favaloro was born in La Plata, Buenos Aires, Argentina, on 14 July 1923. His father Juan B. Favaloro was a carpenter and his mother Ida a dressmaker. Both were Sicilian immigrants. Favaloro grew up in a poor neighbourhood of La Plata and was influenced by his maternal grandmother, who taught him to appreciate nature and the environment, and by his uncle, who was a general practitioner. He often accompanied his uncle on daily rounds in the neighbourhood, which awakened his social conscience and led him towards a career in medicine. He began his studies in the Medical Science faculty of La Plata University, receiving a Bachelor's degree in 1941. After this he served with the Argentine army during World War II. Following discharge as a Lieutenant in 1946, he resumed his medical studies at La Plata, graduating top of his class in 1949.

During his studies, Favaloro was influenced by two of the great Argentinian masters of surgery, Professors Frederico Christman and José Maria Mainetti, who provided an insight into thoracic surgery. He then served an internship at the Polyclinic Hospital in La Plata. At the end of this internship he applied for a position as auxiliary house doctor, was appointed but had second thoughts when asked to write a statement that he accepted the Government's health policy as endorsed by the Peronist party. He stated, 'I began to understand that my future was cloudy because in order to grow and prosper I would have to accept ideas and concepts which were absolutely distant from my previous formation and my spirit.' Favaloro soon resigned because of his intellectual principles, and went to work as a rural surgeon in Jasinto Arauz, a very poor village 300 miles from La Plata. He wrote, 'In total there were maybe 2,000 people when taking into account the rural surroundings. Here one has to do everything from internal medicine to paediatrics, obstetrics, emergency traumatology and minor surgery. Nobody could pay either the physician or the hospital. The money they earned was not enough, even to buy the prescribed remedies.'[1]

As a country doctor, Favaloro branched into other fields, experimenting with preventive medicine, teaching his patients the basic rules of hygiene and organising a group of blood donors in the locality. He knew where each donor lived and called them in as needed. He gradually transformed his own house into a clinic with beds for hospitalisation, X-ray equipment and a small operating room. He was joined by his brother Juan José, who also became a surgeon. They handled all surgical emergencies, developing the practice to undertake gastrectomies, colectomies, oesophageal surgery and gynaecology. Over the next 12 years he broadened his own experience and interest in thoracic surgery, against the background of emerging cardiac surgery occurring in North America and Europe. Exciting news about developments in open heart surgery inspired him to consult his old teacher Dr Mainetti who suggested a fellowship at the Cleveland Clinic. With few resources and rudimentary English, he travelled to Cleveland with the specific view of training in cardiac surgery, then returning to Argentina to treat his fellow countrymen. In the meantime he married his high school sweetheart Maria Antonia Delgardo. The couple had no children.

6.2 The Origins of Coronary Artery Surgery

'Few things are more distressing to a physician than to stand beside a suffering patient who is anxiously looking to him for that relief of pain which he feels utterly unable to afford. Perhaps there is no class of case in which such occurrences as these take place frequently as in some kinds of cardiac disease in which angina pectoris forms at once the most prominent and most painful and distressing symptom.' These were the words of Lauder Brunton from his manuscript on the use of nitrate of amyl in angina pectoris, published in the *Lancet* in 1867.

The range of symptoms and events attributable to coronary artery disease were defined by James Herrick of Chicago in 1912. Differentiation between a prolonged angina attack and acute myocardial infarction was difficult until electrocardiography came into general use in the 1920s. Having identified the association between angina pectoris and coronary atheroma, the next step was to define an appropriate method of treatment. Charles Mayo, co-founder of the Mayo Clinic, first performed cervical sympathectomy for angina in a US Army Major in 1913. During the 1920s, different forms of surgical sympathectomy were undertaken and alcohol was injected into the upper thoracic sympathetic ganglia or nerve roots. Around two thirds of patients were relieved of their angina pain though the natural history of coronary disease progressed inexorably. Efforts to reduce cardiac workload and oxygen consumption began when Elliott Cutler of Boston performed sub-total thyroidectomy for this purpose in 1927. Thyroidectomy was said to provide symptomatic relief in 80% of patients, though they were often transformed into a myxodematous, vegetative existence. Some physicians such as Sir James McKenzie considered that angina symptoms should not be relieved, so as to prevent physical exertion and ventricular fibrillation.

The concept that myocardial blood flow might be increased by surgery began with Claude Beck, Professor of Neurosurgery at the Western Reserve School of Medicine, Cleveland. He sought to boost myocardial blood supply by creating collateral circulation within the pericardium.[2] In 1935, Grosse and Blom at Mount Sinai Hospital, New York, observed that the severity of anginal pain was reduced when the patient developed right heart failure. They argued that congested myocardium had sluggish blood flow from which more oxygen could be extracted. Beck then decided to combine partial occlusion of the coronary sinus with abrasion of the epicardium and pericardium to promote vascular adhesion formation.

Direct attempts to improve myocardial blood flow directly began with Arthur Vineberg at McGill University in 1950. He implanted the left internal thoracic artery directly into the left ventricular myocardium.[3] By three years post-operatively, the first patient was transformed from severe disability through angina to being able to walk 10 miles. In 1964, Vineberg reported 140 operations with 33% mortality but with reproducible relief of angina in those who survived. In 1955, Sydney Smith of Florida modified the Vineberg technique by harvesting the long saphenous vein from the leg and anastomosing the proximal end to the aorta. He then pulled the substance of the vein graft through anterolateral myocardium from base to apex. Again the debilitated patient was asymptomatic 18 months later despite this unlikely solution.

6.3 At the Cleveland Clinic

Two important events occurred immediately before Favaloro's arrival at the Cleveland Clinic. On 5 January 1962 Donald Effler successfully operated on a severe obstruction of the left main coronary artery using a patch graft technique proposed by Ake Senning in Sweden.[4] However, without direct visualisation of the diseased vessels, effective myocardial revascularisation remained only a remote possibility. Selective coronary angiography came about in Cleveland through an almost catastrophic accident. Mason Sones, the radiologist, had introduced techniques for right and left ventricular catheterisation in congenital heart disease which were subsequently used in adults with valvular heart disease. Sones was the first to combine cardiac catheterisation, selective angiography and high speed X-ray motion photography as a single procedure. Serendipitously, on 30 October 1958 Sones was performing a left ventriculogram and had pulled the catheter back into the aorta. As was customary he and his assistant Royston Lewis paused for a cigarette whilst the injector was being re-loaded with 40 ml of contrast agent. He intended to perform an aortogram but the catheter flipped into the right coronary artery before he turned on the camera. The full 40 ml of contrast medium was injected directly into a large right coronary artery which was visualised superbly with all its branches. However, the patient experienced asystole for seven seconds. As Sones recounted, 'I was sure he was going to die and when I looked over at the oscilloscope the ECG was flat. The guy's heart just wasn't beating at all. Well, I knew there was plenty of blood in the aorta so I yelled "cough", figuring that this would push blood into the right coronary and force out the dye. The guy coughed three or four times and his heart resumed beating. There were no defibrillators then. Direct current countershock developed at about the same time and ensured the safety of this technique.'[1]

Sones then designed a special tapered coronary catheter for dependable manipulation. His discovery and refinement of selective angiography could not have been better timed. It defined the pathology of coronary artery disease and contributed to an understanding of the natural history of atherosclerosis. By providing an accurate diagnosis, together with pictures that a surgeon could understand, it proved to be the stimulus for the development of meaningful coronary artery surgery. To quote Floyd Loop, cardiac surgeon and subsequently President of the Cleveland Clinic, 'collectively, all of the cardiological advances in this century pale in comparison with his priceless achievement'. Subsequently, in 1983, Sones (Fig. 6.1) was

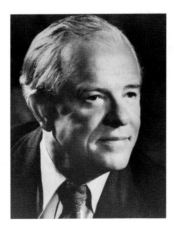

Fig. 6.1. F. Mason Sones Jr (1918–1985). (Courtesy of the Albert & Mary Lasker Foundation.)

awarded the Lasker Clinical Research Award 'for combining the techniques of cardiac catheterization and coronary artery cinematography, thus inaugurating the modern era of diagnosis and treatment of coronary artery disease'.

In the early 1960s, selective coronary angiography was carried out and if a major branch of the left coronary was occluded, the left internal thoracic artery was implanted directly into the ischaemic muscle of this territory. If the right coronary was diseased, the right internal thoracic artery was implanted. If both vessels were occluded, bilateral Vineberg procedures were performed. Despite this, a leading article in the *British Medical Journal* (*BMJ*) in 1967 concluded that 'no operation has yet been shown to increase the patient's expectation of life'.

The ability to study the pathological anatomy of the coronary arteries by cine angiography was the springboard for Favaloro's coronary bypass procedures, though others had attempted direct coronary revascularisation before. In 1953, Gordon Murray had resected the diseased part of a left anterior descending coronary in five patients and replaced it with a vascular graft. He had used the internal thoracic, the axillary or the carotid artery as a graft. Charles Bailey of Philadelphia carried out the first human coronary endarterectomy on 29 October 1956 by incising a right coronary artery beyond the blockage and passing a curette retrogradely through the vessel. The 51-year-old patient was given heparin to prevent thrombosis and made a satisfactory recovery. Encouraged by this, Bailey performed seven similar operations without cardiopulmonary bypass and with symptomatic improvement in each case. Thus, coronary endarterectomy or segmental excision with a saphenous vein or internal thoracic artery graft were performed in the late-1950s before cardiopulmonary bypass came into widespread use. Longmire recalls the first direct anastomosis between the left internal thoracic artery and the right coronary artery in 1958. 'At the time we were doing the coronary thrombo-endarterectomy procedure and we also performed a couple of the earliest internal thoracic to coronary anastomoses. We were forced into it when the coronary artery we were endarterectomising disintegrated and in desperation we anastomosed the left internal thoracic artery to the distal end of the right coronary artery and later decided it was a good operation.'[5]

David Sabiston first employed aorto-coronary saphenous vein bypass in 1962 during a re-operation. He made an end-to-end vein graft to right coronary artery anastomosis. Unfortunately, the patient died three days later from cerebral complications. Probably the first successful saphenous vein bypass graft was by Edward Garrett in 1964 whilst he was working with Michael DeBakey in Houston. He used the vein graft to assist weaning from cardiopulmonary bypass after a prolonged ischemic period. The use and outcome of this procedure were not reported in the literature until 10 years later.

6.4 Favaloro and Sones

At the Cleveland Clinic, Favaloro developed a special relationship with Sones which ultimately led to the development of coronary bypass surgery as a reproducible technique. Favaloro initially had difficulties with the regulatory authorities in the US and could only be accepted as an observer without payment. Donald Effler cut through the red tape and put Favaloro to work in his unit. At the time, the Department of Thoracic Surgery consisted of Effler with his partner Harry Groves and a senior and junior resident. Most of the routine work was lung or oesophageal surgery. Only three or four open heart operations were performed each week. Favaloro began in the intensive care unit and helped clean, siliconise and assemble the enormous heart/lung machine and K-cross oxygenator. From the beginning he also spent time with the radiologists Sones and Shirey, who by then had performed hundreds of coronary angiograms with a degree of precision exclusive to the Cleveland Clinic.[6]

After a few months it became clear to Favaloro that coronary patients fell into two groups: those with diffuse disease that involved most of the coronary branches and those with localised obstruction mainly in the proximal segment but with good distal runoff. By 1964 he passed the Educational Council Foreign Medical Graduate examination and became Chief Resident at the Clinic. When median sternotomy became the standard approach for most heart operations,

Favaloro had the idea that both internal thoracic arteries could be implanted by the Vineberg method. He discussed the idea with Sones who intuitively suggested that necrosis might occur if the sternum was deprived of that blood supply. Reviewing the anatomy he wrote, 'I thought it logical to think this a senseless warning.'

Finally in 1966 (by that time a staff member in the department), Favaloro dissected both internal thoracic arteries and implanted them in the left ventricle. He went on to perform 38 consecutive bilateral implants without mortality or significant morbidity, possibly because the patients were very carefully selected. The assistants at these operations soon grew tired of manually retracting the sternal edges so Favaloro designed his self-retaining retractor. Late re-studies of Favaloro's modification of the Vineberg procedure showed many patients existing on coronary collateral systems with both implants patent. In contrast, a parallel series of patch graft operations on the left main stem carried substantial mortality (11 deaths in 14 patients), so much so that the kidney transplant team asked if they could cross match these patients as prospective donors before surgery.

Early experience with saphenous vein femoro-popliteal bypasses and renal artery reconstructions at the Clinic led Favaloro to think that if saphenous vein grafts worked in the distal circulation, why not in the coronary arteries? In May 1967, the cardiologist David Ferguson referred a 51-year-old woman who had suffered typical angina pectoris for three years. Coronary angiography showed that the right coronary artery was totally occluded in its proximal third. The left coronary was normal and through collateral filling the distal portion of the right coronary appeared patent. Sones and Favaloro decided to begin with this patient since failure of the reconstruction was unlikely to result in fatality. On 7 May, Favaloro resected the occluded portion of the artery and performed a saphenous vein inter-position graft.[7] Angiography eight days later showed excellent flow in the resected vessel. Re-catheterised 10 years later the graft and right coronary artery were still patent. After a few operations using inter-posed saphenous grafts the technique proved troublesome and he turned to the concept of aorto-coronary saphenous vein bypass grafts. Bypass from the antero-lateral wall of the ascending aorta to the end of a resected segment using end-to-end anastomosis was attempted in 15 patients. This was then changed to the simpler end-to-side anastomosis to the coronary artery distal to the blockage. This soon became the enduring technique.

Further substantial advances took place in 1968. Aorto-coronary bypass with saphenous vein was applied to the left coronary artery. The first operation was performed on a patient with severe obstruction of the left main stem but minimal disease in the left anterior descending and circumflex branches. A single vein graft to the proximal left anterior descending coronary showed excellent perfusion of the entire left coronary tree on post-operative angiography. Coronary bypass was then combined with left ventricular aneurysmectomy and valve replacement. By the end of 1968 Favaloro had accumulated a series of 171 patients with single graft direct myocardial revascularisation. After that first year, double then triple bypass procedures followed rapidly. Although, as Sones said, '20th-century cardiology could be divided into the pre-Favaloro and the post-Favaloro era', it was difficult for Favaloro to persuade his colleagues. He persisted in spite of their lack of confidence and the disbelief expressed at different national meetings. Some simply did not believe the low operative mortality (below 5%) and their scepticism led them to question the validity of the statistics.

Direct anastomosis of the internal thoracic artery to an obstructed left anterior descending coronary artery was described by Kolessov in 1967 and then by George E. Green in 1968. In the meantime, Favaloro proceeded to apply coronary bypass in acute myocardial infarction when it became apparent that early restoration of blood flow could limit infarct size. Within a year Favaloro and Sones reported urgent revascularisation in 29 acute infarctions in the *American Journal of Cardiology*. They showed that when revascularisation was achieved within six hours of onset, most of the heart muscle could be preserved.

In 1970, Favaloro was invited to attend the 6th World Congress of Cardiology in London. Donald Ross persuaded him to perform coronary bypass surgery at the National Heart Hospital during this visit. During the operation the scrub nurse accidently pulled the vein off and tore the vessel. At least she did not drop the vein! During this Congress a delegation from Argentina asked Favaloro to return home. This was his original intention, and in October he wrote a letter of resignation to Effler pointing out that his work could be continued by their outstanding residents, Loop and Chalit Cheanvechai. Favaloro's decision to leave Cleveland caused great sadness, particularly to Sones.

When Donald Effler retired from the Cleveland Clinic Floyd Loop became Chief of Cardiac Surgery, and with others, notably Delos Cosgrove and Bruce Lytle, created one of the largest cardiac surgical centres in the world and certainly the best known for research and expertise in coronary bypass surgery. The surgeons persisted with the interrupted suture technique begun by Favaloro. It subsequently transpired that Favaloro's first saphenous vein bypass operation had been preceded by that of Garrett in November 1964, who had tried to perform a patch repair of a localised obstruction in the left anterior descending coronary and resorted to a vein graft because of complications. When Garrett eventually published this case in 1973 thousands of operations had already been performed in Cleveland and other centres in the US.

6.5 Return to Argentina

Irrespective of his prestigious standing and the enormous financial rewards in the US, Favaloro returned to Argentina in 1971. On his departure Dwight Harken of Harvard Medical School commented, 'René, whose love and patriotism to his fatherland made the United States lose one of the world's finest surgeons.'[1] Favaloro (Fig. 6.2) took with him the dream of developing a centre of excellence similar to the Cleveland Clinic for his own country. He understood that such a centre could not exist without research or an efficient educational system. He aimed to raise US$55 million to build the hospital and established the Favaloro Foundation for that purpose in 1975. Favaloro personally financed a research department for the Foundation which evolved into an institute for cardiology, cardiothoracic surgery and organ transplantation with educational influence

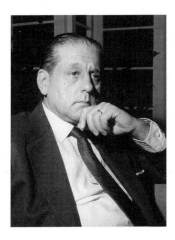

Fig. 6.2. René Favarolo (1923–2000). (http://www.idearia.info/2012/07/homenaje-al-dr-rene-favaloro.html)

all over Latin America. The medical centre and teaching unit were located in the Guemes Private Hospital in Buenos Aires. The Society of Distributors of Newspapers and Magazines donated an eight-storey building as the research centre. The clinic, the Favarolo Foundation Institute of Cardiology and Cardiovascular Surgery, was finally completed in 1992 after which Favaloro developed a television programme called 'The Great Medical Issues', offering information on prevention and treatment of disease. The programme won awards during the mid-1980s. Another television series he created consisted of 24 programmes which focused on the threat of drug misuse in young people.

Increasingly, Favaloro expressed discontent and criticised the state of medicine in Argentina. With the motto 'Advanced technology at the service of medical humanism', the Institute continued to offer specialist services in cardiology and cardiovascular surgery, together with liver, kidney and bone marrow transplantation. Although the hospital treated many private patients, Favaloro continued to focus on the problems of the indigenous poor population on a daily basis, focusing on disease prevention and promotion of basic hygiene to reduce mortality from infectious diseases. Such was the popularity of the hospital that it ran into debt. In a letter to the editor of

La Nacion, a Buenos Aires newspaper, he stated that his foundation was owed $18 million by state-owned hospitals and medical centres.

In 2000, Argentina had been in depression for two years and was submerged in an economic and political crisis. By now the Favaloro Foundation was in debt by US$75 million. Favaloro petitioned the Argentine Government to aid the hospital but never received an official response. He personally wrote to President Fernando De La Rua, asking for help to clear the Foundation's debts, but apparently the letter was never read. At one meeting he commented that 'we are without doubt submerged in a materialistic, hypocritical and dehumanised society that has been developing slowly but steadily and which appears to have no limits to its appetites. All means are justified to increase power and pressure through economic gains. It is of no importance that the greatest part of the population is excluded and survives in misery and lack of welfare'. Weeks before his death Favaloro wrote, 'I am going through the saddest period of my life. In the most recent times I have been turned into a beggar.'[8] This referred to the increasingly difficult task of finding enough money to provide medicines or surgery for the poor.

On 29 July 2000 Favaloro shot himself through the heart at his home in Buenos Aires. Whether suicide was a deliberate statement against the state of the world in which he had to beg for money to cure people or whether it was simply the act of someone desperately sad was difficult to decide. Inevitably the financial ruin of his medical centre was the precipitating factor. In Favaloro's honour the President declared 31 July 2000 'a national day of mourning in recognition of Favaloro's deep love and attachment to his country'.

6.6 Conclusion

Undoubtedly Favaloro deserved this recognition for his humanitarian approach to medical care in Argentina. Whether he deserved a Nobel Prize for the development of coronary bypass surgery is another matter. History shows that he was not the first surgeon to perform aorto-coronary bypass, but in the words of Sir Francis Darwin, 'in science the credit goes to the man who convinces the world not the man to whom the idea first occurs'.[9] This comment is perhaps best exemplified in the giants of cardiac surgery. The legacy of Favaloro was summarised in an essay by Bernard Lown who stated:

> In 1967 the Argentine surgeon Dr Rene Favaloro working at the Cleveland Clinic, successfully used a vein graft to bypass an obstructive coronary vessel. Like Edmund Hillary and Tensing Norgay, the first climbers to reach the summit of Mount Everest, or Roger Bannister, the first to run a 4-minute mile, Favaloro opened a terrain deemed beyond human reach. In coronary surgery he sundered the barrier to the seemingly impossible.[10]

Within 10 years, 100,000 patients were helped by coronary bypass operations in the US. By the 1990s the number had quadrupled and Favoloro's efforts had transformed cardiac surgery worldwide. In the author's view a Nobel Prize shared between Sones and Favoloro would have been appropriate, given the significance of their pioneering work which addressed the principle cause of death in the Western world.

References

1. Westaby S. Surgery for coronary artery disease. In: Westaby S and Bosher C (eds), *Landmarks in Cardiac Surgery*. Oxford: Isis Medical Media; 1997: pp. 187–221.
2. Beck CS. The development of a new blood supply to the heart by operation. *Ann Surg* 1935; 102: 801–813.
3. Vineberg A, Miller G. Internal mammary coronary anastomosis in the surgical treatment of coronary artery insufficiency. *Canad Med Assoc J* 1951; 64: 204–210.
4. Effler DB, Sones FM Jr, Favoloro RG, Groves LK. Coronary endarterectomy with patch graft reconstruction: clinical experience with 34 cases. *Ann Surg* 1965; 162: 590–597.
5. Longmire WP Jr, Cannon JA, Kattus AA. Direct-vision coronary endarterectomy for angina pectoris. *N Engl J Med* 1958; 259: 993–999.
6. Sones FM Jr, Shirey EK. Cine coronary arteriography. *Mod Concepts Cardiovasc Dis* 1962; 31: 735–738.

7. Favoloro RG. Saphenous vein autograft replacement of severe segmental coronary artery occlusion. *Ann Thorac Surg* 1968; 5: 334–339.
8. Letter to *La Nación*, Argentina (no publication details available).
9. Darwin, F. Francis Galton. *Eugen Rev* 1914; 6: 1–17.
10. http://bernardlown.wordpress.com/2012/03/10/mavericks-lonely-path-in-cardiology (Accessed: 31 July 2013).

Chapter 7

CHRISTIAAN BARNARD AND NORMAN SHUMWAY: THE HEART TRANSPLANT PIONEERS

Stephen Westaby and David Marais

7.1 Background to Cardiac Transplantation

"Thus sayeth the Lord God, a new heart also will I give you, and a new spirit will I put within you; and I will take away the stony heart out of your flesh, and I will give you a heart of flesh" (Ezekiel, Chapter 36 verse 26).

Aristotle considered the heart to be the seat of the soul. This concept prevailed well into the 20th century and provided ethical constraints on the scientific discussion of cardiac transplantation.[1] By 1905 Charles Guthrie and Alexis Carrel had perfected microvascular suture techniques and transplanted allograft hearts into the necks of recipient animals. They recognised that the rapid destruction of the grafted tissue was due to a toxic effect of the host's blood on the transplanted organ. It was not until 1944 that Peter Medawar showed that rejection of skin grafts was due to an immunological reaction and that the same applied to transplanted organs. The stimulus for renal transplantation began with the remarkable achievements of Willem Kolff, who developed renal dialysis during the Nazi occupation of Holland in 1944 (See Chapter 13). Cardiac transplant animal models were originally employed to study the effects of drugs such as thyroxine on the denervated heart. In 1933 Frank Mann of Rochester, Minnesota, transplanted canine hearts into the carotid jugular circulation. He emphasised the importance of restoring the coronary artery circulation as quickly as possible. If reperfusion was delayed the heart muscle lost its tone and the valves failed to function. In successful experiments cardiac action started at once with a constant rate of between 100 and 130 beats per minute. Mann's longest-surviving canine transplant recipient lasted for eight days. Histological examination of the excised heart showed mottling and ecchymosis, infiltration with lymphocytes, large mononuclear cells and neutrophils. Mann postulated that a biological factor was the cause of death and correctly described the cytological basis of acute organ rejection.

Clinical interest in cardiac transplantation began in 1951 when Marcus, Wong and Luisada at Chicago Medical School reported their experience with a modified Mann preparation:

> The problem which we are attempting to explore can be stated as follows: Can a combination of highly specialised tissues, the heart, be grafted in a mammalian animal? Can such a graft live in a homologous environment? Can such a graft actually function by receiving and delivering blood? Whether it might so function as to replace its counterpart in the host is a matter of fantastic speculation for the future![2]

Meanwhile unbeknown to the West, Vladimir Demikhov performed many remarkable transplant experiments at the Moscow State University. In 1946 he transplanted hearts into the thorax of dogs as an auxiliary pump. Between 1946 and 1958 he carried out 250 experiments in 24 different ways. His aim was to determine the best vascular connections to achieve adequate filling of both sides of the transplanted heart. Demikhov had no heart/lung machine but with two animals lying side by side he used rubber tubes and temporary anastomoses in such a way that a cardiac transplant could be carried out without interrupting the circulation to either the recipient animal or the donor organs. In 1951, after 67 operations, he achieved a post-operative survival of six days. As well as cardiac transplantation Demikhov transplanted puppies' heads on to the necks of adult dogs. The transplanted heads apparently reacted normally to their surroundings and would lap up water when thirsty. Because of language and other barriers, Demikhov's work was unknown to the West until 1962 when his book was translated into English. David Wheatley, Professor of Cardiac Surgery in Glasgow and a student in Cape Town in 1962, recalls sitting in the surgeons' changing room when a report of Demikhov's head transplant appeared in the Cape Argos newspaper. The news was conveyed to Christiaan Barnard who was clearly put out. He stormed out with the retort that 'anything those Russians can do, we can do too'. That same afternoon Barnard transplanted the head of a dog onto a recipient dog, which survived for several days. Animal rights protestors were incensed and the medical students built a papier mâché two-headed dog for their Rag Parade. Barnard had already walked the tightrope between genius and vulgarity.

For orthotopic cardiac transplantation a simplified surgical method was required to avoid multiple anastomoses of pulmonary veins and vena cava. In 1952, Cookson, Neptune and Bailey were able to use systemic hypothermia to stop an animal's circulation completely for 30 minutes without harm. In 1957, Webb and Howard reported on 'restoration of function of the refrigerated heart'. They demonstrated that canine hearts heparinised and flushed with potassium citrate could survive for prolonged periods at low temperature (4°C) and subsequently regain function when transplanted heterotopically. Anticipating long distance heart procurement, Webb and Howard commented that when the problem of immunology was solved, it would presumably take several hours to obtain the heart, prepare the recipient and perform re-implantation. Consequently their methods for myocardial protection seemed to render clinical cardiac transplantation feasible.

7.1.1 *Cardiopulmonary bypass*

The introduction of cardiopulmonary bypass by Gibbon in 1955 greatly increased the feasibility of transplantation. In Puerto Rico a group led by Blanco, the head of Bailey's research laboratory, employed a pump oxygenator to sustain the transplant recipient and potassium citrate arrest of the donor heart during the ischemic period. After restoring coronary blood flow the transplanted heart began to beat vigorously. Again failure occurred within days through rejection. In 1958, Goldberg, Berman and Akman at the University of Maryland reported on three experimental orthotopic cardiac transplants. Their major contribution was to transect the left atrium in order to circumvent the need to individually anastomose the pulmonary veins. In 1959, Webb, Howard and Nielly accomplished 12 successful orthotopic transplants using hypothermia to preserve the donor heart and the pump oxygenator to maintain the recipient. Also in 1959 Ross and Brock of Guy's Hospital in London described six different methods of cardiac excision and replacement. They used both right and left atrial cuffs to reduce the multiple pulmonary venous and vena caval anastomoses down to two atrial anastomoses.

The following year Lower and Shumway published the cardinal paper on orthotopic cardiac transplantation in which advances in surgical technique, recipient support and donor organ preservation were integrated into a single approach.[3] Of eight consecutive dog transplants, five recipients survived between six and 21 days. All were functionally restored to eat and exercise. This was the first description of a simple and reproducibly successful technique for mammalian orthotopic cardiac transplantation that enabled recipient animals to return to normal activity. No immunosuppressive agents were used so death occurred from rejection and rapid myocardial failure. Histology showed massive infiltration by lymphocytes and interstitial haemorrhage. Lower and Shumway then proposed that if the host immunological system could be prevented from destroying the heart in all likelihood it would continue to function adequately for the normal life span of the animal.

7.1.2 *Immunosuppressive therapy*

It was the advent of immunosuppressive therapy for renal transplantation which proved the key to clinical cardiac transplantation. Keith Reemtsma of Tulane University School of Medicine increased the survival time for cardiac allografts in the neck from 10 days in untreated animals to 27 days for those who received methotrexate at the onset of rejection. In 1964 he performed heterotopic transplants with elective azathioprine immunosuppression after which the treated animals lived for up to 32 days. In contrast, Adrian Kantrovitz and co-workers at Maimonides Hospital, Brooklyn, performed orthotopic transplants in three-month-old puppies and achieved survival times of up to 213 days without any immunosuppression. Kantrovitz noted that long-term survivors showed no histological evidence of rejection and grew steadily with time. This was encouraging information for the eventual application of heart transplants in infants. By 1967 Richard Lower, now at the University of Virginia, described survival up to 15 months for orthotopic transplanted hearts in dogs using methotrexate. A transplanted bitch even gave birth to a litter of healthy puppies, the father of which also had a heart transplant. Lower and Shumway used the prolonged survival of human renal transplant recipients to justify their cardiac allograft programme. Shumway commented, 'enough has been achieved in fact to provoke expression of the concept that only the immunological barrier lies between this day and a radical new era in the treatment of cardiac diseases'.[1]

7.1.3 *Xenotransplants*

By 1964, the first human cardiac transplant had already taken place, at the University of Mississippi Medical Center, Jackson. However, the first human recipient did not receive a human heart. Hardy was expecting the donor heart to be obtained from a young patient dying of traumatic brain injury for a recipient with terminal ischemic heart failure. The key issue was how soon after cardiac standstill could the donor heart be removed. In an attempt to avert irreversible ischaemic damage to the transplanted heart, Hardy planned to insert catheters into the donor femoral vessels and begin total body perfusion as soon as death was pronounced. The timing of donor heart removal did not include the concept of brain death — only cardiorespiratory arrest constituted legal demise. Consequently unless the donor's clinicians were willing to suspend ventilator support it was exceedingly unlikely that a potential donor would die within the time limits during which the recipient could reasonably be kept alive on the heart-lung machine. Hardy had spent many years in basic animal research and had performed mock operations on human cadavers so that his team was prepared. He had performed the first human lung transplant in 1963 and gained experience with immunosuppressive drugs and cobalt radiotherapy. With the knowledge that primate kidneys had been used for renal xenotransplantation Hardy had confidence that a chimpanzee heart would provide suitable back up should the logistics of human transplantation fail.

The patient was a 68-year-old man with hypertension and lower leg gangrene. He had been admitted pulseless and comatose but was resuscitated. Further management included tracheostomy, mechanical ventilation, femoral embolectomy and below knee amputation. Elsewhere in the hospital a young patient was dying of irreversible brain damage but not quickly enough to save the potential recipient. Eventually the prospective recipient went into cardiogenic shock but the prospective donor had not yet deteriorated to the state where death was imminent. The patient was placed on cardiopulmonary bypass and a 44 kg chimpanzee anaesthetised in an adjacent operating room. Shumway's transplant guidelines were used, apart from the fact that the donor heart preservation was achieved by retrograde coronary sinus perfusion with chilled oxygenated blood. The transplant was technically satisfactory but the chimpanzee's heart was unable to maintain the recipient's circulation. He died approximately one hour after discontinuing cardiopulmonary bypass.

In 1966, Lower performed mirror image experiments of Hardy's transplant whereby human hearts were resuscitated following donor kidney removal and then implanted into baboons. In one such experiment the resuscitated human heart provided satisfactory circulatory support in the baboon for several hours. This was never reported in the medical literature but Shumway and others were aware of Lower's experiments. These confirmed that a heart could be stopped, removed, resuscitated and successfully transplanted. By the summer of 1967 Shumway felt that the three most crucial issues with cardiac transplantation had been solved. In an interview for the *Journal of the American Medical Association*, he stated that 'the time was right for human heart transplantation, if a potential recipient and compatible donor could be found simultaneously'.[1] In fact Shumway had a 35-year-old man with end stage cardiac disease in hospital awaiting transplantation at the time. The patient had undergone extensive radiotherapy for Hodgkin's disease and already had a depressed immunological system. The interview was published in November and shortly afterwards Kantrovitz in New York sent out 500 telegrams to other medical centres in search of a donor. However, it was Christiaan Barnard who was first past the post with his transplant on 9 December 1967.[4]

7.2 Biography of Christiaan Barnard

Christiaan Barnard was born on 8 November 1922 in a small South African town, Beaufort West (population around 10,000 people). His father served as a minister and despite the relative poverty of the area, was able to raise his children well whilst serving a mixed race community. Christiaan was the fourth child in the family. The first born studied engineering, the second pregnancy yielded a still-born twin sister and the third a blue baby who died at the age of two, presumably from Fallot's Tetralogy. Four years after Christiaan, his brother Marius was born and was also destined for a surgical career. At school Christiaan was intelligent, well-motivated and determined to achieve. He then studied medicine at the University of Cape Town with a curriculum strongly influenced by British medical schools. A surgical career seemed unlikely when he found the initial exposure to human dissection and autopsies challenging. He fainted when he assisted a general practitioner at an appendicectomy in his home town.

Immediately after qualifying Barnard worked temporarily as a general practitioner in Namibia, then as a houseman for Professor Crichton in gynaecology in Cape Town. He then joined a general practice in Ceres, a village 120 km from Cape Town and while there he married an operating theatre sister Louwtjie, whom he had met during his student years. He then returned to a post in infectious disease medicine in Cape Town (1951–1953) which led to a thesis on the treatment of tuberculous meningitis. Barnard's interest then switched to surgery. He joined the academic department at Groote Schuur Hospital where he worked on various animal models with Professor Jannie Louw. One of these models involved hypothermic surgery on the heart.

Witnessing Barnard's orientation towards experimentation and an academic career, Professor J. F. Brock steered him towards a fellowship in thoracic surgery at the University of Minnesota, under the direction of Professor O. H. Wangensteen. In Minneapolis he was assigned to the oesophageal group but was soon drawn towards the pioneering work of Walton Lillehei and Richard De Wall, who were developing a heart-lung machine. At the time there were only two hospitals in the world performing open heart surgery: the Mayo Clinic and the University of Minnesota Medical Center. These were only 90 miles apart. Visitors from all parts of the world travelled to both institutions to observe their methods. With his experimental background Barnard saw the potential of using a pump oxygenator to perfuse organs for transplant.

Barnard returned to South Africa in 1958, joining Groote Schuur Hospital as a cardiothoracic surgeon and the University of Cape Town as lecturer and Director of Surgical Research under Professor Louw. Before Barnard left the University of Minnesota, Wangensteen, in recognition of his enthusiasm, made a telephone call to the National Institutes of Health to request a $2000 grant for a heart-lung machine for him to take back to South Africa together with $2000 per year for three years of experimental work. With this pump Barnard progressed steadily towards a clinical organ transplantation programme. In 1960 he transplanted a second head onto a dog and visited the Soviet Union to discuss other transplants. He also began paediatric cardiac surgery with his anaesthetist Dr Ozinsky who remained with him to supervise cardiopulmonary bypass.

By 1963 Barnard began to explore cardiac transplantation in dogs. He practised the Lower and Shumway technique to preserve the atrial walls and intra-atrial septum in the recipient. Clinical renal transplants were being undertaken by Dr David Hume in Richmond, Virginia, where Richard Lower was also practising transplantation of animal hearts at the Medical College of Virginia. Understanding the importance of managing organ rejection, Barnard first spent three months at the renal unit at Richmond then visited Thomas Starzl in Denver, who was beginning to use the immunosuppressant, antilymphocyte serum. Returning to Cape Town in September 1967 Barnard performed a human renal transplant in a patient who subsequently lived for more than 20 years. After 48 technically successful dog heart transplants and in the knowledge that Shumway and Lower had a 90% success rate in more than 300 transplanted dogs, Barnard was now satisfied that a human heart could be transplanted with minimal risk.

7.3 Biography of Norman Shumway

Norman Shumway Jr was born on 9 February 1923 to Norman Edward Shumway and Laura Irene Van der Vliet who ran the dairy in his home town of Jackson, Michigan. He excelled at high school and was a key member of the debating team which won the State debating contest. He then entered the University of Michigan in September 1941, initially for a pre-law degree but he also took classes in engineering. When drafted into the Army, his colonel gave him the choice of the infantry, medicine or dentistry as career alternatives. Shumway was quick to select medicine and was despatched to Waco, Texas, to complete an accelerated pre-med course. From there he transferred to Vanderbilt University in 1945 from which he graduated in medicine in 1949. He spent a summer elective at the Massachusetts General Hospital and was impressed by hearing about the new operations for cardiovascular disease being performed at the University of Minnesota. He applied for and was awarded a surgical residency there in 1949. The first two years were spent in general surgery after which he was called up for Air Force service during the Korean war.

On returning to Minneapolis he spent two years working towards a PhD on hypothermia to facilitate open heart surgery with F. John Lewis. Dr Wangensteen was head of the department and strongly supportive of the exciting developments in cardiac surgery achieved by Lillehei, Varco and colleagues.

Shumway married Mary Lou Stuurmans in 1956. Upon completing his surgical residency and declining a post in the cardiovascular service, the Shumways travelled to Santa Barbara, California. Here Shumway joined an older partner in private practice and performed one of the first open heart operations in California. This was successful but the combination of a senior and conservative thoracic surgeon with a young raconteur was not a good match. Six weeks later Shumway was fired for what was called 'gross insubordination'. He then took a post at Stanford University Medical School performing haemodialysis but by then the Shumway family had grown to include four children and it was necessary to find a more lucrative job.

It was in the rustic conditions of the research laboratory at Stanford where the early work on topical cooling for myocardial preservation and transplantation took place. Assisting in the laboratory was the young resident Richard Lower. In 1958, when the Medical School moved to Palo Alto, Shumway by default became the only cardiac surgeon at the Stanford Campus. By now the University of Minnesota had awarded him a PhD for his thesis entitled 'Experimental surgery of the heart and great vessels under hypothermia (PhD 1956)'. Thus, having declined Chief Residency with Wangensteen's service to undertake private practice, he switched back to an academic post at the University of California, San Francisco. Leon Goldman, the Chief of Surgery, fell asleep during Shumway's interview but he was nonetheless hired to run the kidney dialysis machine at Stanford Lane Hospital. He was also asked to operate the heart-lung machine with Dr Roy Cohn at the Children's Hospital. With Raymond Stofer, Shumway worked out an extraordinarily simple perfusion system with a minimum of gauges and monitors to clean or repair. Simplicity soon became the hallmark of Shumway's surgical advances.

When Stanford Lane Hospital moved to Palo Alto and became the Stanford University Medical School, Shumway became Professor and Chairman of the Department of Cardiovascular Surgery (1974). Shumway wrote:

> When I started work at Stanford the idea of cardiac transplantation grew out of our local cooling experiments since we had one hour of aortic cross clamping during cardiopulmonary bypass. Accordingly we decided to remove the heart at the atrial level and then to suture it back into position. After several of these experiments, we found it would be easier to remove the heart of another dog and do the actual allotransplant. Something like 20–30 experiments were performed before we had a survivor. All of this was done before chemical immunosuppression was available.[1]

Lower presented their early work at the 'Surgical Forum' in 1960.[3] It was an early morning talk and only the projectionist, the moderator and Drs Shumway and Lower were present. Work continued in the laboratory whilst clinical correction of congenital heart disease began at the Palo Alto campus. One of the earliest series was of patients with Fallot's Tetralogy. They found that these patients did better with topical cooling of the heart in the operating room. When Lower took his oral Boards in Thoracic Surgery, he described 100 Fallot's Tetralogy operations without a death. The examiner thought that he was making it up. After a dog named Ralphie had survived for a year with another dog's heart Shumway expressed an opinion that human heart transplantation was imminent. By then Lower had taken an appointment at the Medical College of Virginia and was continuing his transplant research in the laboratory. Inadvertently he became the umbilical cord connecting Barnard and Shumway (Fig. 7.1) to provide the setting for which most believed would be the first clinical cardiac transplant.

7.4 The First Human Heart Transplant

In 1967, South African law allowed organ removal when a donor was declared dead by two doctors, one of whom should have been quali-

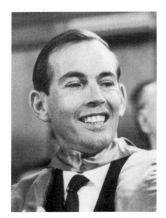
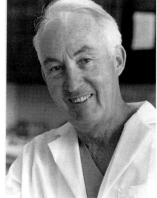

Fig. 7.1. Christiaan Barnard, left, in academic gown. (Courtesy of the Transplant Museum, Groote Schuur Hospital). Norman Shumway, right. (Office of Communication and Public Affairs, Stanford School of Medicine.)

fied for more than five years. Neither of the doctors could be involved in the transplant team. Legally the mode of death need not be defined and it was possible to use the concept of irreversible brain injury. Permission was required from either the relatives or the Coroner. Undoubtedly Barnard was well prepared for the operation. He chose as a potential recipient Louis Washkansky who had end stage ischaemic cardiomyopathy. Washkansky's angiograms had already been sent to the Cleveland Clinic for an opinion on the feasibility of coronary bypass surgery but he had been deemed inoperable. This approach was different from the US where surgeons anticipated cardiac transplantation for an on-table surgical failure. The Barnard team decided not to use either a black donor or recipient because of potential criticism. The recipient's signed consent form, where his name is misspelt Waskansky, is shown in Fig. 7.2.

The donor for the first transplant was a 25-year-old machinist Denise Anne Darvall. She was shopping with her mother in Cape Town when a car left the road and hit both women. Mrs Darvall was killed immediately. Denise sustained serious head injuries and was first admitted to a local hospital, resuscitated and then transferred to the neurosurgeons at Groote Schuur Hospital. Washkansky was a 54-year-old diabetic with three previous extensive myocardial infarctions and intractable heart failure. In reality he was a poor candidate. He had diabetes, gross ascities due to right heart failure and *Pseudomonas* cellulitis where metal Southey's cannulas had been inserted into the groin to drain oedema. However donor and recipient's blood groups were compatible and Denise had a similar leucocyte antigen pattern to Washkansky's.

In the early hours of 3 December 1967, Washkansky was taken to the operating theatre, anaesthetised and his chest was opened. Examination of the heart suggested that nothing other than transplantation could help him. Meanwhile, when a neurosurgeon stated that Denise's brain injuries were irrecoverable, she was taken to the adjoining operating theatre. Her ventilator was disconnected and as soon as the heart fibrillated, supportive cardiopulmonary bypass and cooling were established by femoral cannulation. Body temperature was reduced to 26°C. Sternotomy was performed, the aorta clamped

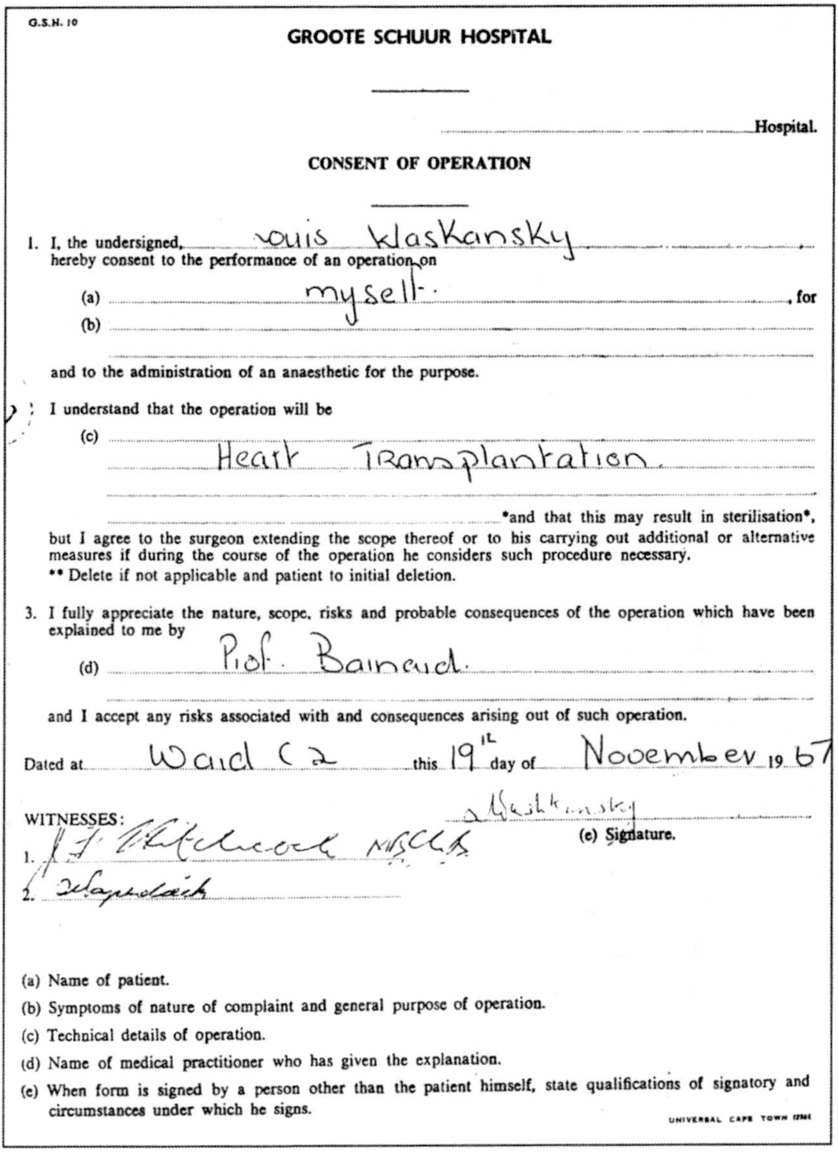

G.S.H. 10

GROOTE SCHUUR HOSPITAL

....Hospital.

CONSENT OF OPERATION

1. I, the undersigned, ...Louis Klaskansky........
hereby consent to the performance of an operation on

(a) ....myself...................., for

(b) ....

and to the administration of an anaesthetic for the purpose.

I understand that the operation will be

(c) ....Heart Transplantation...................

....*and that this may result in sterilisation*,
but I agree to the surgeon extending the scope thereof or to his carrying out additional or alternative
measures if during the course of the operation he considers such procedure necessary.
** Delete if not applicable and patient to initial deletion.

3. I fully appreciate the nature, scope, risks and probable consequences of the operation which have been
explained to me by

(d) ....Prof. Barnard...................

and I accept any risks associated with and consequences arising out of such operation.

Dated at........Ward C2........this 19ᴸ day of........November 19 67

WITNESSES:

1. ....L. Klaskansky........
(e) Signature.

2. ....

(a) Name of patient.
(b) Symptoms of nature of complaint and general purpose of operation.
(c) Technical details of operation.
(d) Name of medical practitioner who has given the explanation.
(e) When form is signed by a person other than the patient himself, state qualifications of signatory and
circumstances under which he signs.

UNIVERSAL CAPE TOWN 27ME

Fig. 7.2. Consent to the first human heart transplant, signed two weeks
pre-operatively.

and the heart cooled to 16°C. It was then excised and placed in a bowl of physiological saline at 10°C. The beating heart was transferred to the adjacent operating room and reperfused with blood after only four minutes. Meanwhile, Washkansky was placed on cardiopulmonary bypass but the arterial line pressure in the diseased femoral vessel was very high. Barnard, assisted by Terry O'Donovan and Roger Hewitson, decided to transfer the cannula to the ascending aorta. In the excitement of the moment they clamped the arterial line without stopping the bypass machine. When disconnected it sprayed blood throughout the whole operating room. Air was pumped when the system was reconnected and worse still the sino-atrial node of the donor heart was damaged by ligation of the superior vena cava-right atrial junction. The donor heart required pacing and it took three attempts to wean it from cardiopulmonary bypass. Nevertheless the operation was completed successfully.

The donor heart had arrived in the operating room at 3 a.m. and by 6.15 a.m. the operation was concluded with a satisfactory cardiac output. The Medical Superintendent of the hospital was informed of the event some time later with the short sentence, 'Sir, we have just transplanted a heart and the patient is well.'

Washkansky's post-operative care was meticulous. Immunosuppression was started on the day of surgery with corticosteroids and azathioprine. Cobalt irradiation was applied to the heart on the fifth, seventh and ninth post-operative days. He was kept in isolation within the same operating room in order to minimise the infection risk. In practice it was difficult just to keep the reporters out. Washkansky's response to the transplant was remarkable (Fig. 7.3). Signs of heart failure soon disappeared after a substantial diuresis. His grossly oedematous legs returned to their normal shape by the third post-operative day and the swollen liver involuted to normal size. Diabetes was easier to control.

Inevitably, the media response was enormous, massively intrusive and not always complimentary. In a BBC broadcast the interviewer asked Barnard whether he had performed the transplant to improve the bad image of South Africa. Americans inferred that Barnard had stolen both the idea and surgical methods from Shumway. This was

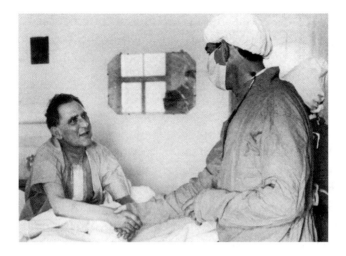

Fig. 7.3. Grateful patient shakes hands with Barnard after the operation.

inappropriate because the principles and methods of cardiac transplantation had been published in medical journals and Barnard had performed numerous animal experiments in preparation. Three days after the Washkansky operation, Adrian Kantrowitz found an anencephalic infant donor and transplanted its heart into a two-day-old baby. This was a nine-hour operation and the tiny recipient died on the operating table.

Two weeks after the transplant Washkansky showed signs of either pneumonia or rejection of the transplanted heart. Despite antibiotics and steroids the situation worsened and caused his death on 21 December. The heart maintained a good cardiac output until the last moment. The post-mortem findings were reported in the *Lancet* by James Thompson, Professor of Pathology at Groote Schuur Hospital:

> Necropsy on the first heart transplantation in man confirmed that death was due to extensive bilateral pneumonia and not to rejection of the heart. Signs of rejection, however, were demonstrated histologically but were of a low order compared to those seen in the transplanted dog heart. How far the mildness of the rejection signs is to be ascribed to species differences, immunosuppressive drugs and procedures, post-operative rest and nursing and medical care or to the good matching of leukocyte antigens cannot at the moment be assessed.[5]

Even before Washkansky's death, an international panel of prominent cardiac surgeons was convened in the Plaza Hotel, New York, to discuss the ethical implications. Bailey, who in the early 1950s had caused controversy in his hospital by his rush to perform a successful mitral valvotomy, declared the South African transplant to be 10 years premature. Jacob Zimmerman, a colleague of Bailey's at New York's St Barnabas Hospital agreed, adding, 'it is medically and morally wrong for doctors to stand by a dying patient's bedside hoping he will get it over with quickly so we can grab his heart'.[1] In contrast, Donald Ross, a fellow South African and former classmate of Barnard's, and the Swiss surgeon Ake Senning both said that they would perform transplants and they were optimistic that heart banks would be established where organs could be stored. In Houston, Michael DeBakey established his own committee to deliberate the question and concluded that heart transplants were as yet untenable. On learning of this decision his great rival Denton Cooley, in the neighbouring Texas Heart Institute, re-doubled his own efforts to find a donor.

Barnard's operation aroused hostility in the US because it appeared to pre-empt Shumway's careful and systematic work published since 1959. The profession complained that the immunological difficulties had not been resolved, that Barnard's first human transplant was premature, flamboyant and irresponsible. James Hardy, who transplanted the chimpanzee's heart to man in 1965, reflected the chagrin of many Americans:

> I confess my disappointment was enormous though not so much for myself personally, for I knew that Shumway's group at Stanford had done the most extensive and best work in the field. We had long been waiting for them to transplant a heart in man following which we planned to transplant another.[1]

Some, including Cooley, Kantrovitz, DeBakey and even Shumway were more generous. DeBakey stated:

> Barnard has broken the ice. It is a real breakthrough in the whole field of heart replacement. It is a great achievement. There were at least 20 medical centres in the world where there was skill and knowledge enough to perform

transplants. What we have all been waiting for is the right circumstances — the right donor and the right recipient. Dr Barnard had the right circumstances and he did it. They took the first step, we will do it too.[1]

7.5 Subsequent Human Heart Transplants

Barnard was encouraged by the first transplant and not perturbed by the fatal outcome. On 2 January 1968, he transplanted a heart into a 58-year-old Cape Town dentist named Philip Blaiberg. On this occasion the donor was a 24-year-old factory worker who had suffered a massive sub-arachnoid haemorrhage whilst sunbathing on a Cape Town beach. When his condition was declared hopeless he was transferred from Victoria Hospital to Groot Schuur Hospital pending the transplant. The operation transformed Blaiberg from a breathless cardiac cripple into an independent man able to drive a car and swim in the sea. He spent 73 days in hospital but then lived for 18 months before dying from chronic rejection.

On 6 January 1968, four days after the Blaiberg transplant, Shumway transplanted the heart of 43-year-old Virginia May White into a 54-year-old steel worker, Mike Casparak. Mrs White had collapsed with a cerebral haemorrhage whilst celebrating her 22nd wedding anniversary and Casparak was dying from chronic viral myocarditis. Misfortune dogged the operation from the start. The diseased heart was so large that the pericardial cavity was almost three times the size of the donor organ. This resulted in technical problems, and five hours post-operatively Casparak was returned to the operating room with bleeding and cardiac tamponade. Two days later his liver and kidneys failed and he suffered diffuse gastrointestinal bleeding. He required a vast volume of transfused blood (288 pints at a total cost of $7,200) and then peritoneal dialysis. On the eighth post-operative day he underwent cholecystectomy under local anaesthesia but lapsed into hepatic coma and died on 21 January. The hospital bill for this operation was $28,845, almost $2,000 a day for the 15 post-operative days. This expenditure brought about a barrage of criticism from many who felt that the money could have been better spent.

Kantrovitz attempted a further paediatric transplant three days after the Casparak operation. This operation lasted for nine hours, the patient survived for six hours only and Kantrovitz withdrew from the transplant scene. Shortly afterwards, Sen in Bombay lost a transplant patient on the operating table and Cabrol in Paris transplanted a truck driver who died without regaining consciousness. Donald Ross at the National Heart Hospital, London, and Denton Cooley at St Luke's in Houston, performed their first transplants on 3 May 1968. Ross's operation was undertaken on 45-year-old Frederick West, who was hospitalised with chronic severe congestive heart failure. The previous day, a 26-year-old building worker had sustained serious head injuries during a fall and despite craniotomy at King's College Hospital could not be saved. When Ross was told about the donor, the body was rushed across London in an ambulance with the circulation sustained by external cardiac massage (see Chapter 8). West survived for 45 days.

Cooley's first patient was 47-year-old Everett Thomas who had been bedridden for five months with rheumatic heart disease and needed triple valve replacement. He also had paralysis and blindness following cerebral emboli. Valve surgery was scheduled for 3 May but two days beforehand a 15-year-old female with a gunshot wound to the brain was referred as a transplant donor. Coincidentally, Cooley had operated on her coarctation of the aorta at the age of nine and she still had a hypertrophied left ventricle. Cooley explained to Thomas and his family that the chances of surviving triple valve replacement were small and that a potential heart donor was available. He suggested valve replacement initially, but cardiac transplantation should Thomas not be able to be weaned from cardiopulmonary bypass. The donor and potential recipient were moved to adjacent operating rooms and when it was established that Thomas's heart was irreparable, Cooley's colleague Grady Hallman harvested the donor heart. No cooling or myocardial protection were used. The detached heart continued to beat and was implanted directly with 35 minutes ischaemic time.

The heart functioned well and within 72 hours Cooley had performed two further transplants. The next donor was the 15-year-old son of a personal friend of Cooley and the recipient a hospital administrator whose cardiac problem had been deemed inoperable a few months earlier. By the middle of August 1968 Cooley had performed nine transplants, but despite large numbers of accidents and homicides in Houston, donors were scarce. St Luke's Hospital and surrounding motels soon overflowed with patients awaiting urgent transplants and on one occasion Cooley transplanted a sheep's heart into a 48-year-old man. This rejected acutely and fatally on the operating table without giving time for re-replacement with a pig's heart. On 17 August Cooley transplanted the heart of an 8-year-old boy with severe head injuries into a 5-year-old girl with congenital heart disease. She survived for less than a week.

7.6 Consequent Events

The front page of the Cape Argos newspaper on Monday 4 December 1967 showed a picture of Washkansky recovering in the intensive care unit, a picture of the donor Denise Darvall with the headline, 'They will miss Denise', and a leading article reporting the three years of laboratory research which preceded the operation. Between Barnard's first and second transplant, he travelled to the US for media interviews but was not well received by the American surgeons. From a personal standpoint, Barnard achieved superstar status with worldwide public acclaim. His cardiac surgeon brother Marius, who made significant contributions to the research and early operations, acknowledged that Christiaan was fundamentally changed by his celebrity status. This was to lead to divorce from his first wife and further marriages and divorces. Sadly his son, who had qualified in medicine and specialised in paediatrics, took his own life.

The technical details of cardiac transplantation were not difficult to master, but logistical problems prevented progress. Fundamental to the transplant process was the concept and definition of brain death. Failure to resolve this issue proved problematic. Shumway commented: 'It should be underlined that no-one can transplant a dead heart. The hearts which have been transplanted by surgeons all over the world could have been resuscitated in the donors and the chests could have been closed leaving these hopelessly brain injured persons to the fate of infection or peripheral vascular collapse. Death of the donor is a diagnosis which must be made by the neurological and neurosurgical team.'[1] This concept was fundamental to transplantation of all organs. Heart transplantation continued at Groote Schuur Hospital and a building was erected to promote the work in 1972. This attracted many foreign doctors to study cardiac surgery in Cape Town. Whilst Barnard maintained an interest in research work, international fame impacted on his ability to continue a clinical programme. He was said to have developed significant problems with rheumatoid arthritis and was self-conscious about plastic surgery for skin cancer. This, together with demoralisation after his son's suicide, led to his retirement from cardiac surgery in 1983. Perhaps inadvisedly, he transferred his interests to cosmetic surgery and preventing the ravages of advancing age. He retired to Switzerland, and after living in relative obscurity he died unexpectedly from an asthma attack in Cyprus at the age of 78.

Though initial outcomes were discouraging, the advent of clinical cardiac transplantation was a stimulus for Shumway. During the 12 months after Barnard's first operation over 100 transplants were performed in almost 50 different centres. Almost 60% of the patients had died within 10 days, with a mean survival of <30 days. Amongst the medical profession enthusiasm waned rapidly and the number of operations decreased. Most physicians considered that the procedure should be limited to hospitals with a record of transplant research and a successful renal transplant programme. Such departments could provide tissue typing and immunosuppressive therapy together with strategies to prevent infection and rejection. These criteria favoured Shumway's unit at Stanford, Lower's unit at Richmond, Virginia, and both the Texas Heart Institute and Baylor. The most significant advance in anti-rejection therapy came with the introduction of transvenous endomyocardial biopsy by Philip Caves in 1972.[6] Caves, who came from Glasgow, worked as a research fellow at Stanford and devised a bio-tome (Konno had already produced such a device in Japan) which was introduced through the right internal jugular vein. This was advanced to the right ventricle of the transplanted heart to obtain a biopsy. Another Stanford innovation was the introduction of T-cell monitoring and anti-thymocycte globulin. Then followed the introduction of cyclosporin A following research by Roy Calne and colleagues in Cambridge. With significant improvements in organ preservation and anti-rejection therapy, the Registry of the International Society for Heart Transplantation in 1988 showed 2,450 heart transplants by 118 centres in the US, 61 in Europe and 23 in other parts of the world. Hospital mortality fell below 10% whilst five years actuarial survival increased to almost 75%. Centres carrying out more than 50 transplants a year showed lower mortality figures and patients treated with cyclosporin A, azathioprine and steroids had a five-year survival of 80%. Shumway's carefully followed cardiac transplants continued and outdistanced all other series in number, quality of results and yield of scientific information. Without Shumway's persistence and scientific efforts cardiac transplantation could easily have been abandoned.

Shumway retired from his role as Chief of Cardiovascular Surgery at Stanford University on 9 February 1993. Almost all of his trainees returned to mark the event. During the ensuing 30 years of semi-retirement he continued to operate intermittently, travelled to international meetings and enjoyed offering advice. He is known for several sayings, including 'all bleeding stops', 'air rises' and 'there is plenty of time for sleep on the other side of the grave'. He died in 2006.[7]

7.7 Conclusion

In retrospect, did the development of cardiac transplantation warrant a Nobel Prize? If so, should this have been awarded to Barnard, who undertook the clinical risk in a forgiving environment, or to Shumway for his translational research and persistence? Perhaps to both, jointly. In effect, outcomes in the first few years were not encouraging and more recently the procedure has been described as 'epidemiologically trivial'.[8] In other words, the achievement was more spectacular than clinically important. Perhaps apartheid and the political situation in South Africa were also a deterrent, though this proves ironic for a hospital and university that were opposed to apartheid and for a surgeon who grew up in a family that directly served the indigenous community.

References

1. Westaby S. The beginnings of cardiac transplantation. In: Westaby S and Bosher C (eds), *Landmarks in Cardiac Surgery*. Oxford: Isis Medical Media; 1997: pp. 253–277.
2. Marcus E, Wong SN, Luisada AA. Homologous heart grafts; transplantation of the heart in dogs. *Surg Forum* 1951; 1: 212–217.
3. Lower RR, Shumway NE. Studies on orthotopichomo transplantation of the canine heart. *Surg Forum* 1960; 11: 18–19.
4. Barnard CN. The operation. A human cardiac transplant: an interim report of a successful operation performed at Groote Schuur Hospital, Cape Town. *S Afr Med J* 1967; 30 December: 1271–1274.
5. Thompson, JG. Heart transplantation in man — necropsy findings. *Br Med J* 1968; 2: 511–517.
6. Caves PK, Stinson EB, Billingham ME *et al*. Diagnosis of human cardiac allograft rejection by serial cardiac biopsy. *J Thorac Cardiovasc Surg* 1973; 66: 461–466.
7. Shumway SJ. A Tribute to Norman E Shumway MD, PhD 1923–2006. *Heart Failure Clin* 2007; 3: 111–115.
8. Eric Rose cited in http://www.harthosp.org/transplant/Heart Transplantation/HeartTransplantinPerspective/default.aspx (Accessed: 28 July 2013).

Chapter 8

WILLIAM KOUWENHOVEN AND PAUL ZOLL: THE INTRODUCTION OF EXTERNAL CARDIAC MASSAGE, DEFIBRILLATORS AND PACEMAKERS

Max Lab

8.1 Introduction

Up until 2011, 199 men had been awarded the Nobel Prize in Physiology or Medicine and only 10 women, which presumably reflects the paucity of women in science in the earlier years. Gerti Cori was the first woman to win it, in 1947, together with her husband Carl Ferdinand Cori, 'for the discovery of the course of the catalytic conversion of glycogen', and they shared it with Bernardo Houssay, 'for his discovery of the part played by the hormone of the anterior pituitary lobe in the metabolism of sugar'. As with the women who struggled to succeed in the Nobel stakes there were also men who lost out in this event. The specific example to be considered here is cardiac resuscitation, and the two men concerned were William Kouwenhoven and Paul Zoll.

Why should Kouwenhoven and Zoll have earned the Nobel Prize? Their thoughts were preceded in 1930 by Albert S. Hyman in humans (but also, in animal experiments, by Steiner in 1871, Greene in 1872 and Ziemssen in 1882).[1] With his engineer trained brother, Hyman had constructed and patented an 'artificial pacemaker': a crank-handle turned a spring motor to turn a magnetic DC current generator.

When the device was used in New York, the medical community rejected it, while others deemed the process unnatural. Kouwenhoven's and Zoll's work was also preceded in 1949 by John Hopps, an engineer. Canadian medical researchers working on hypothermia approached him because they found that hypothermic hearts went in to asystole, and rewarming them was too slow a process to restore normal rhythm. Hopps designed and constructed a catheter electrode for venous introduction, in order to atrially stimulate the heart in experimental animals with a vacuum tube-operated external pacemaker.

However, Kouwenhoven and Zoll saw further. One supposes they could invoke the saying *'If I have seen further it is by standing on ye shoulders of Giants'* — an aphorism attributed to Isaac Newton's letters, but really ascribed to Bernard of Chartres in the 12th century. Thus, Kouwenhoven developed external cardiac massage as well as open- and closed-chest defibrillators. External cardiac massage is simple, needing no clinical instruments, and is used to sustain the circulation after a variety of cardiac pathological onslaughts. Zoll devised the closed-chest defibrillator and the pacemaker[2] — life-saving instruments serving to prevent sudden and random death. Thousands of patients have benefited from these procedures, and thousands of patients worldwide have received pacemakers. The latter need continues, with thousands more implanted year on year.

8.1.1 *Brief biographical sketches*

Wiliam Kouwenhoven was born in Brooklyn, New York, in 1986 and became Professor of Electrical Engineering at the Johns Hopkins School of Engineering in 1914. In 1928, the Edison Electric Company decided to fund research into the sudden deaths by electrocution of several of their linemen. Despite his lack of any medical training, Kouwenhoven's research from then on was focused on the effects of electricity on the heart and in 1933 his laboratory showed that an electrical shock could stop ventricular fibrillation in dogs. He went on to show that a shock could also revive the human heart, and thus pioneered the concept that electric shocks could reverse ventricular fibrillation.

Kouwenhoven was Dean of the Engineering Faculty at Johns Hopkins from 1938 to 1954 and in 1969 he received the first honorary degree ever bestowed by the Johns Hopkins University School of Medicine. Together with Zoll (Fig. 8.1) he received the Lasker Clinical Research Award in 1973 'for his life-saving development of open- and closed-chest defibrillators, and for originating the technique of external cardiac massage'. He died in 1975.

Paul Zoll was born in Boston in 1911. He obtained his medical degree from Harvard Medical School and then worked as a cardiologist at the Beth Israel Hospital in Boston for the remainder of his career. In 1952, he demonstrated that application of alternating current electric shocks via external electrodes placed on the chest could stimulate an asystolic heart to beat. He went on to develop the notion of continuous monitoring of cardiac rhythm, now used routinely in every coronary care unit, and he also invented the cardiac pacemaker, a modern cardiologist's indispensable tool. He shared the Lasker Award with William Kouwenhoven in 1973 'for his development of the life-saving closed-chest defibrillator and the pacemaker'. He died in 1999.

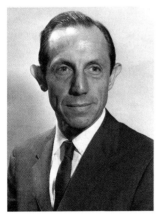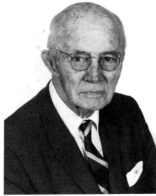

Fig. 8.1. Paul Zoll and William Kouwenhoven. (Courtesy of the Albert and Mary Lasker Foundation.)

8.2 Some of their Instrumentation

William Kouwenhoven developed instruments for open- as well as closed-chest defibrillation, but there was still the problem of patient management during the interval before access to a defibrillator. To this end he devised and instituted external cardiac massage, which maintained an effective circulation to sustain patients until they reached hospital facilities. Patients with ventricular fibrillation are as effectively in cardiac standstill as are those in pure cardiac arrest. Unusually (and perhaps hopefully for some of the authors of this book), he developed these concepts when more than 68-years-old and after his retirement in 1954. Although anyone can apply this relatively simple manoeuvre, it is best to have had training, as do ambulance personnel, the police and firefighters, as well as those attending recognised first aid courses. Further work showed that cardiopulmonary resuscitation (CPR) by machine-operated external compression (Fig. 8.2 a)[3] was superior to manual compression[4] and Zoll designed, built and patented a portable CPR system (Fig. 8.2 b).[5]

Paul Zoll also pioneered electrical techniques in cardiology: in 1952 he showed that externally applied electric stimulation could restart the heart, and later showed that it can defibrillate it, as well as curtailing other life-threatening rhythm disturbances. Continually

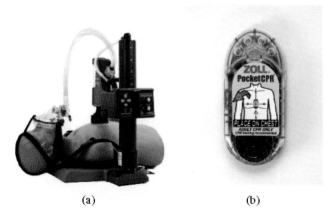

(a)   (b)

Fig. 8.2. Early instruments for pacing and resuscitation. a. Hands-free CPR system.[3] b. The portable CPR device designed by Zoll.[5]

perfecting his defibrillator, in 1958 Kouwenhoven completed a closed-chest defibrillator. It was an independent and parallel contribution to Paul Zoll's, who additionally researched the theoretical and technical approaches to cardiac rhythm monitoring with its clinical application, adopted by coronary care units. He also instituted technical training modules in resuscitation.[5]

8.3 A Slant to their Studies — A Cardiac Electromechanical Yin–Yang

There is a kind of Chinese philosophical Yin–Yang (or Yin and Yang) related to the overall work of William Kouwenhoven and Paul Zoll. Yin–Yang translates as 'shadow and light', where seemingly opposite ideas or notions are interconnected and interdependent (Fig. 8.3). They are not opposing but interact in a greater dynamic system. For example, one cannot fully understand shadow without light. Yin and Yang do not imply evil and good. This section treats Kouwenhoven's and Zoll's research in the cardiopulmonary field as a kind of Yin–Yang in death, with opposing resuscitation.

8.3.1 *Electrical Yin — electrically-induced resuscitation*

In contrast to the fatal effects of an electric shock described below (Section 8.3.2) Kouwenhoven later found, in open-chested dogs, that a roughly similar electrical shock could have the opposite effect — it could restart hearts (Fig. 8.3, top). In the 1940s this was exploited as a therapeutic manoeuvre in humans, and Kouwenhoven developed a defibrillating device that could pass a current to the heart through the chest wall. Medical research at that time took second place to World War II, but after the war, Kouwenhoven's researchers completed this device — a small container with its cables connected to copper paddles. The hospital to which Kouwenhoven was attached (Johns Hopkins) exploited the device in cardiac arrest. Surmising that he could produce an instrument that could electrically reach the heart through the chest, much research after World War II produced a defibrillator by around 1957. Users began to treat cardiac arrest by

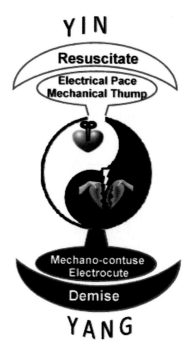

YIN

Resuscitate

Electrical Pace
Mechanical Thump

Mechano-contuse
Electrocute

Demise

YANG

Fig. 8.3. A Yin–Yang approach to Zoll and Kouwenhoven's electromechanical research. Central is the iconic Yin–Yang symbol. The top heart within the icon is the resuscitated heart, functioning normally — like clockwork. The Yin: electrically, one can pace the heart. Mechanically one can also pace, but in addition resuscitate by mechanical CPR, and thump version. The bottom (split) heart is electromechanically compromised, for as opposed to the top, we have Yang. We can electrocute, and a thump can kill.

applying a couple of copper paddle electrodes from a relatively small electronic box.

8.3.2 *Electrical Yang — death*

About a century ago, it was first noticed that a relatively small electrical shock could kill, immediately (Fig. 8.3, bottom). But Kouwenhoven wondered otherwise and took advantage of the Edison Electric Company's research support into the 'electro-physiological' consequences of electricity on the body (the company men working on the lines were being electrocuted!). Although around the 1920s they had found that large shocks had terminal cardiorespiratory effects, for example in experimental rats, there then came mechanically-induced resuscitation.

8.4 Mechanical Yin — Mechanically-induced Resuscitation

8.4.1 *Mechanical pacemaker*

Eduard Schott first described percussion pacing, a procedure that is not well known despite it being quickly instituted and easy for emergency cardiac pacing.[6] International and European Clinical Committees on Resuscitation recommend it in their support guidelines (Nolan and colleagues).[7] However, Paul Zoll later[8] put percussion pacing 'on the map' with his mechanical thumper. Figure 8.4 shows a patient whose cardiac output was non-existent, but then shows activating ECG complexes with each mechanical percussion. Cessation of percussion shows records with no complexes.

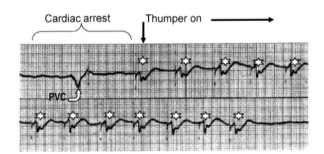

Fig. 8.4. ECG from patient with cardiac arrest with percussion pacing. The patient was in cardiac arrest, with only occasional premature ventricular complexes (PVC) seen. On starting percussion (thumper on) each chest tap activated the heart with each producing an ECG complex. Cardiac standstill was seen as soon as percussion stopped. (Modified from *N Engl J Med*, Zoll P. M., Belgard A. H., Weintraub M. J. *et al.*, External mechanical cardiac stimulation, 294, 1274–1275, copyright Massachusetts Medical Society. Reprinted with permission from Massachusetts Medical Society.)

8.4.2 *Mechanical cardioverter: thump version*[9-11]

A mechanical thump to the front of the chest is a quick resuscitative procedure in an emergency and can cardiovert ventricular fibrillation. It is safe, and a chest thump should be given early, followed by CPR. Guidelines recommend those trained in the technique to attempt thump version.

In an Italian study, a cardiac monitor was connected to suspected victims during a thump before any other interventions. Heart rhythm, circulation, hospital discharge and adverse effects were monitored. No adverse effects on heart rhythm were observed and when thump version failed, so did other procedures. Mechanical resuscitation was also used as a pacemaker — a mechanical thumper. However, the acidosis associated with delay of the thump (say, in hospital versus out of hospital) renders this less successful, or it can even be detrimental.[12]

8.4.3 *Mechanical cardiopulmonary resuscitation*

William Kouwenhoven's laboratory later observed that using the heavy paddles of the defibrillator to push on the chest raised blood pressure, and this was carefully tested in the operating theatre. They found that not only was blood pressure raised with chest compression, but repetitive compression of an arrested heart circulated blood — enough for vital oxygenation, albeit a bit less than half normal. Combining this with mouth-to-mouth resuscitation eventually led to cardiopulmonary resuscitation, now abbreviated to CPR. More recently this procedure has been developed and a CPR device has been constructed (see, for example, Fig. 8.2 a) and proved to be more effective than manual CPR.[4,13]

8.4.4 *Mechanical cough cardioversion*[14-16]

A study of the value of precordial thumps and of cough cardioversion outside hospital, showed that mechanical intervention was successful in cardioverting ventricular tachyarrhythmias. Repeated coughing can keep individuals conscious for up to a minute's duration. Coughing compresses the heart and can sometimes produce arterial pressure waves greater than external chest compression. Cough cardiac compression (i.e. by oneself) does little to traumatise the chest wall or heart and is not position-related, as is external compression, and could be life-saving (see Chapter 6).

8.5 Mechanical Yang — Mechanically-induced Death

8.5.1 *Commotio cordis*[17–21]

Commotio cordis is often described as concussion of the heart through a blunt object's blow to the area of chest over the heart (Fig. 8.5). The impact does not penetrate the chest, nor does it produce structural damage, but is followed by sudden death from

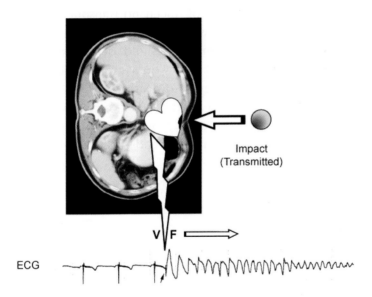

Fig. 8.5. Diagram depicting *commotio cordis*, with chest impact by blunt object producing no cardiac damage, but inducing ventricular fibrillation (VF). The diagrammatic heart is in the centre of the chest (radiographic cross section.) The blunt object (ball) strikes the front of the chest, the transmitted impact temporarily distorting the heart surface and producing VF (lower ECG). A dramatic example of this sequence of events during a karate bout is shown in a video posted on YouTube (http://www.youtube.com/watch?v=LLtzT2bXVGI).

ventricular fibrillation. It can, but not necessarily, be related to underlying cardiac abnormality.[22] It is a leading cause of sudden cardiac death in young athletes.

The electrophysiological consequences of blunt force trauma were determined to be critically dependent on the timing of the impact within a 20-millisecond window, 10–30 milliseconds before the peak of the T-wave. The velocity (>40 mph) and the hardness of the impacting object directly relate to the initiation of ventricular fibrillation.[23]

8.6 The Mechanisms behind Kouwenhoven's and Zoll's Work

Initially, the mechanisms of these findings were unknown but have now been revealed as a variant of 'mechano transduction', probably stretch activated channels[24–27] where mechanical deformation of the cardiac membranes can produce threshold depolarisation. This is capable of activating the heart and would explain the resuscitating mechanical thumper (a Yin) but also death by *commotio cordis* (the Yang), probably by activation of the kATP mechano-sensitive ion channel.[28,29] The impact produces a pro-arrhythmic current between cells within the cardiac deformation, and those within the normal areas.

8.7 Current State-of-the-Art Implantable Pacemakers and Defibrillators

Modern pacemakers are implanted subcutaneously below the clavicle with their electrodes traversing the subclavian vein until they reach their locations in the right atrium and ventricle. They emit low energy electrical pulses to overcome both brady- and tachyarrythmias and to suppress atrial fibrillation. They also have the ability to record and store electrocardiographic information concerning cardiac rhythm and function.

A more recent development is the implantable cardioverter-defibrillator (ICD), which is inserted in a similar manner to a pacemaker.

This can not only function as a pacemaker but also has the ability to deliver high-energy electrical pulses so as to counteract potentially fatal arrhythmias such as ventricular fibrillation and *torsade de pointes* in patients with the long QT syndrome.

The most recent development is the subcutaneous ICD (S-ICD) which can deliver enough electrical energy through the chest wall to revert ventricular fibrillation to normal rhythm without the need for intracardiac electrodes. This device was recently approved by the FDA for use in the US.

8.8 Conclusion

In an analogous manner to Kolff's and Scribner's life-saving contributions to clinical nephrology so too have Kouwenhoven's and Zoll's inventions saved countless lives and radically influenced cardiological practice. And it is not just clinicians who have benefited from their work, it is also lay members of the public faced with dealing with a cardiac arrest in the street or at the office. Without doubt, these pioneers enhanced the Yin and diminished the Yang of electrically-mediated cardiac events. However, as discussed in Chapter 13 in relation to haemodialysis, there may be a perception among some academics that Kouwenhoven's and Zoll's findings were not sufficiently groundbreaking in scientific terms to merit a Nobel Prize. Be that as it may, the practical impact of their discoveries was summed up by the late Michael DeBakey, legendary cardiac surgeon and chairman of the jury that gave them their Lasker Award: 'Until the work of these two men, there was just no way of dealing with a heart emergency.'[30]

References

1. Geddes LA, Moore CR. Stimulation with electrosurgical current. *Australas Phys Eng Sci Med* 1990; 13: 63–66.
2. Zoll PM, Linenthal AJ, Norman LR *et al*. Use of external electric pacemaker in cardiac arrest. *J Am Med Assoc* 1955; 159: 1428–1431.
3. http://www.michiganinstruments.com/life-stat (Accessed: 1 August 2013).

4. Dickinson ET, Verdile VP, Schneider RM *et al*. Effectiveness of mechanical versus manual chest compressions in out-of-hospital cardiac arrest resuscitation: A pilot study. *Am J Emerg Med* 1998; 16: 289–292.

5. http://www.zoll.com (Accessed: 1 August 2013).

6. Eich C, Bleckmann A, Schwarz SK. Percussion pacing — an almost forgotten procedure for haemodynamically unstable bradycardias? A report of three case studies and review of the literature. *Br J Anaesth* 2007; 98: 429–433.

7. Nolan JP, Deakin CD, Soar J *et al*. European resuscitation council guidelines for resuscitation 2005. Section 4. Adult advanced life support. *Resuscitation* 2005; 67: Suppl 1: S39–S86.

8. Zoll PM, Belgard AH, Weintraub MJ *et al*. External mechanical cardiac stimulation. *N Engl J Med* 1976; 294: 1274–1275.

9. Davis EY. Posterior thump-version. *N Engl J Med* 1971; 284: 919.

10. Pellis T, Kette F, Lovisa D *et al*. Utility of pre-cordial thump for treatment of out of hospital cardiac arrest: A prospective study. *Resuscitation* 2009; 80: 17–23.

11. Pellis T, Kohl P. Extracorporeal cardiac mechanical stimulation: Precordial thump and precordial percussion. *Br Med Bull* 2010; 93: 161–177.

12. Miller J, Tresch D, Horwitz L *et al*. The precordial thump. *Ann Emerg Med* 1984; 13: 791–794.

13. Timerman S, Cardoso LF, Ramires JA *et al*. Improved hemodynamic performance with a novel chest compression device during treatment of in-hospital cardiac arrest. *Resuscitation* 2004; 61: 273–280.

14. Caldwell G, Millar G, Quinn E *et al*. Simple mechanical methods for cardioversion: Defence of the precordial thump and cough version. *Br Med J (Clin Res Ed)* 1985; 291: 627–630.

15. Criley JM, Blaufuss AH, Kissel GL. Cough-induced cardiac compression. Self-administered from of cardiopulmonary resuscitation. *JAMA* 1976; 236: 1246–1250.

16. Criley JM, Blaufuss AH, Kissel GL. Self-administered cardiopulmonary resuscitation by cough-induced cardiac compression. *Trans Am Clin Climatol Assoc* 1976; 87: 138–146.

17. Link MS, Estes NA, III. Mechanically induced ventricular fibrillation (commotio cordis). *Heart Rhythm* 2007; 4: 529–532.

18. Link MS, Wang PJ, Maron BJ *et al.* What is commotio cordis? *Cardiol Rev* 1999; 7: 265–269.
19. Madias C, Maron BJ, Alsheikh-Ali AA *et al.* Commotio cordis. *Indian Pacing Electrophysiol J* 2007; 7: 235–245.
20. Maron BJ, Ahluwalia A, Haas TS *et al.* Global epidemiology and demographics of commotio cordis. *Heart Rhythm* 2011; 8: 1969–1971.
21. Maron BJ, Doerer JJ, Haas TS *et al.* Historical observation on commotio cordis. *Heart Rhythm* 2006; 3: 605–606.
22. Maron BJ, Doerer JJ, Haas TS *et al.* Commotio cordis and the epidemiology of sudden death in competitive lacrosse. *Pediatrics* 2009; 124: 966–971.
23. Maron BJ, Gohman TE, Kyle SB *et al.* Clinical profile and spectrum of commotio cordis. *JAMA* 2002; 287: 1142–1146.
24. Lab MJ. Mechanosensitivity as an integrative system in heart: An audit. *Prog Biophys Mol Biol* 1999; 71: 7–27.
25. Lab MJ, Dean J. Myocardial mechanics and arrhythmia. *J Cardiovasc Pharmacol* 1991; 18: Suppl 2: S72–S79.
26. Sachs F. Stretch-activated ion channels: What are they? *Physiology (Bethesda)* 2010; 25: 50–56.
27. Kohl P. Commotio cordis: Early observation. *Heart* 1999; 82: 397.
28. Garan AR, Maron BJ, Wang PJ *et al.* Role of streptomycin-sensitive stretch-activated channel in chest wall impact induced sudden death (commotio cordis). *J Cardiovasc Electrophysiol* 2005; 16: 433–438.
29. Link MS, Wang PJ, Vander Brink BA *et al.* Selective activation of the K(+)(ATP) channel is a mechanism by which sudden death is produced by low-energy chest-wall impact (commotio cordis). *Circulation* 1999; 100: 413–418.
30. http://www.time.com/time/magazine/article/0,9171,908176,00.html#ixzz2HhrAwbBt (Accessed: 1 August 2013).

Chapter 9

INGE EDLER AND CARL HELLMUTH HERTZ: THE DEVELOPMENT OF ULTRASOUND FOR CLINICAL USE

Bhavna Batohi and Paul S. Sidhu

9.1 Introduction

Ultrasound in medical diagnosis involves the use of high frequency sound waves directed towards an organ. The sound waves are then reflected back when they reach tissues of differing acoustic impedance, thereby forming the basis of the echo principle. Much of the progress of clinical ultrasound ensued from the use of sonar and radar in World War II and the discovery of the piezoelectric effect.[1] Through the collaboration of Inge Edler and Hellmuth Hertz, the acoustical science of cardiology and the physics of the ultrasonic echo method were brought together to create echocardiography. In 1997, the Albert Lasker Clinical Medical Research Award was given to Inge Edler 'for pioneering the clinical application of ultrasound in the medical diagnosis of abnormalities of the heart — probably the most useful non-invasive tool for cardiac diagnosis since the electrocardiograph machine', and to Hellmuth Hertz 'for pioneering the development of ultrasound technology in medicine'.

Their research using ultrasound initially focused on mitral valve disease but through further investigation and experiments they found that other heart conditions could be evaluated with ultrasound.[2] Their innovation stimulated the clinical development and application of ultrasound in other fields including obstetrics and gynaecology, paediatrics, neurology and general radiology, and spawned the development of ultrasound guided interventional and therapeutic procedures.

Although the pair were nominated several times for the Nobel Prize in Medicine, they never achieved this accolade, and in fact the field of medical ultrasound has yet to receive recognition with the award of a Nobel Prize. This non-invasive technique is the second most commonly utilised diagnostic imaging modality after conventional X-rays.[3] Computed tomography (CT) and magnetic resonance imaging (MRI) both secured a Nobel Prize for their inventors despite being far less utilised in medical diagnosis on a worldwide stage. Ultrasound makes a difference to people the world over, is relatively inexpensive, portable and uniquely a 'safe' imaging technique that most importantly has transformed maternal health — ultrasound has saved the lives of countless unborn children.

This chapter details the work of Edler and Hertz, recognised as the pioneers in the medical ultrasound field, and describes how their pioneering work encouraged extensive study into this field, with developments in countless areas by numerous other scientists and clinicians. Recent advances in ultrasound will also be highlighted.

9.2 Brief Biological Sketches

9.2.1 Inge Edler

Inge Edler was born on 17 March 1911 in Burlöv, Malmöhus County, Sweden. Both his parents were teachers. Edler developed a curiosity for technology during his youth and initially intended to study physics but was dissuaded by his sister, who encouraged him to take up a course in dentistry as an alternative. He missed the course application deadline for dentistry and so enrolled to do medicine instead. Edler attended the University of Lund, always planning to remain in medicine only until he could re-apply for dentistry. However, he became intrigued by medicine, stayed on the course and graduated in 1943.[4,5]

From 1944, Edler moved to Malmö, developing his career in internal medicine with an interest in cardiology. In 1948, he became responsible for cardiac catheterisation and angiography and was appointed Director of the Laboratory for Heart Catheterisation in Malmö, later returning to Lund University where he became head of the Department of Cardiology.

Whilst in Lund, Edler worked with Professor Helge Wulff, a pioneer in the field of cardiac surgery and closed mitral valve commisurotomy procedures. Edler appreciated that cardiac catheterisation and contrast imaging was still in its infancy and could not provide sufficient detail on the status of the mitral valve so that there was the necessity for non-invasive pre-operative diagnostic methods.[6] Edler desired to quantify the degree of mitral stenosis in patients prior to open heart surgery in order to determine the existence of mitral insufficiency, a vital consideration.[7] He was familiar with the use of radar and sought to use this echo technology for the benefit of patients.[8]

It was during the 1950s and 1960s that Edler, the clinician, met and worked with Hertz, the scientist, in the development of echocardiography. Edler was considered to be the quieter and more reflective of the duo and practically orientated.[2] His colleagues described him as having 'an ardent interest for the patient, interdisciplinary creative thinking, extreme accuracy coupled with an infinite patience', attributes that made him successful in his research.[6] He was meticulous in the way he carried out his work; information and data received from Edler was always accurate. 'With this concentration on his work, Edler was sometimes regarded as rather correct in an old-fashioned way but also a very kind person. Beneath his official exterior there was always a great amount of humanity, cordiality and sense of humour together with a natural curiosity within many different areas.'[6]

Following his retirement in 1977 Edler utilised his medical knowledge to help biomedical engineering students at Lund Institute of Technology. In 2000, he was awarded the title of 'The Swedish Cardiologist of the 20th Century' by the Swedish Cardiology Society, and is today regarded as the father of echocardiography.[8]

Inge Edler married Karin, had four children and died in 2001, just ten days prior to his 90th birthday. Appendix A is a list of Edler's numerous accomplishments.

9.2.2 Carl Hellmuth Hertz

Hellmuth Hertz was born on 15 October 1920 in Berlin, Germany. His family was well recognised in the world of physics with his uncle, Heinrich Hertz, being the physicist after whom the unit of frequency of radio waves is named. His father, Gustav Hertz, was a physicist too and in 1926 received the Nobel Prize in Physics. During his earlier days, Gustav worked for a light bulb factory in Holland where he was authorised to do basic research and developed the ability to make fluorescent tubes flexible enough to be shaped into different signs and letters, thereby enabling glowing neon tubes to be used in signs for the first time. He patented this idea, and this heralded the use of neon tubes for advertising. The light bulb factory that Hertz worked in is now Philips, the multinational electronics company.[9] Hellmuth's father was great friends with other physicists who very often visited his home, thereby creating an inspirational environment for the young boy (Fig. 9.1).

In 1939, Hertz graduated from Schule Schloss Salem, a boarding school, considered to be one of the most prestigious in Germany. Hertz was due to further his studies at Technische Hochschule, Berlin, but was conscripted into the Armed Forces during World War II and served in North Africa.[9] While in North Africa he was captured and taken prisoner of war by the Americans and transferred to the United States. Hertz originally studied mathematics at the University of Chicago and was awarded a one-year scholarship in 1947 to study physics in the Department of Theoretical Physics at the University of Lund, organised by Niels Bohr and Torsten Gustafsson. While in Lund, Hertz wrote a thesis on the use of ferromagnetic rings as an electronic memory device and designed the first accelerator in the department, the Graff generator. In 1955, Hertz completed a PhD in physics with a thesis on high-voltage corona discharges. He was described as having a 'broad knowledge of fundamental physics and natural inclination for applied physics'.[9] Hertz became more interested in biophysics; however, this enthusiasm for a relatively new field was not shared by his colleagues in the physics laboratory.[9] In 1963, Hertz became Professor of Electrical Measurements at the new

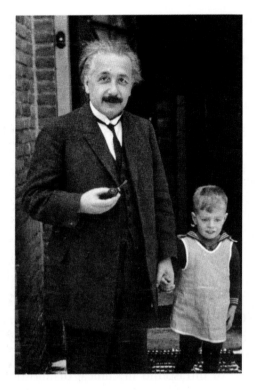

Fig. 9.1. Albert Einstein and Carl Hellmuth Hertz in Germany. (Courtesy of the South Swedish Society for the History of Medicine.)

Institute of Technology in Lund, which was part of the University of Lund.[9]

Hertz was said to be an 'excellent advisor and inspiration to all scientists working in Lund'[9] but did not publish in the scientific literature as widely as expected. Only if an idea was his very own and if he had done the majority of the work himself would he publish the results. As far as possible, Hertz avoided experimenting in fields that others had already discovered in order not to hinder his own thought processes when working on a project. Upon retirement he became the first Emeritus member of the editorial board of *Ultrasound in Medicine and Biology.*[9]

Upon his death in 1990, Hertz was described as having 'exceptional cleverness in creating new and useful inventions', 'endless spontaneous creative spirit', and a 'hard and purposeful procedure to actively create new ideas'.[9] Appendix B is a list of Hertz's various accomplishments.

9.3 Nature of the Scientific Question

In the early 1950s, Edler sought a non-invasive method to quantify the degree of mitral stenosis and determine the presence of mitral insufficiency prior to surgery.[2] He was already familiar with radar as used in World War II and was particularly interested in deploying 'SONAR' (sound navigation and ranging) in pre-surgical diagnosis. Hertz already possessed an interest in biophysics, stimulated by the writings of Ludwig Bergmann in *Der Ultraschall* (1954), detailing the possibilities of SONAR; this encouraged him to consider the use of ultrasound in clinical diagnostics.

Edler and Hertz met after Edler had asked the husband of one of his nurses, Jan Cederlund, a physicist in Lund, if the radar technique could be used to examine the heart and diagnose mitral regurgitation. Cederlund handed the enquiry on to Hertz, who he knew was already exploring the use of ultrasound in clinical diagnostics. At this stage Hertz recognised that radar could not provide a level of resolution adequate for visualising human organs but that by using much higher sound frequencies (MHz) there might be a prospect of achieving this. Hertz got together with Edler and the progressive discovery of the clinical use of ultrasound began in earnest in Lund.[8,10]

9.4 Description of the Research (the 'Discovery')

Pierre and Jacques Curie had completed the discovery of piezoelectricity in 1880.[4] They were both physicists exploring the energy propagation of sound waves and 'observed that an electric potential would be produced when mechanical pressure was exerted on a quartz crystal such as the Rochelle salt (sodium potassium tartrate tetrahydrate)'.[1] During World War II there was development of pulse-echo SONAR which was used to aid underwater detection of objects and also for communication. Floyd A. Firestone at the University of

Michigan and Donald Sproule in England were the early pioneers in the application of pulse-echo equipment for detecting flaws in metals, but this metal flaw detection equipment became accessible to bio-medical researchers only after the war.[11]

In May 1953, after contacting Edler, Hertz went to a shipyard near Malmö where he was aware of an ultrasound 'reflectoscope' that was employed for flaw detection and used to test welding seams in ships.[12] Hertz placed the ultrasound probe on his chest and observed that the generated echo moved in step with his own heart. He borrowed the machine for a weekend and took it to Lund, where he and Edler used it on themselves and patients, and made the initial discovery which would develop into a priceless tool for cardiac diagnosis (Fig. 9.2).

Hertz's father had been director of the Siemens Research Laboratory before the end of the war. This connection enabled Edler and Hertz to secure a long-term loan of a reflectoscope from the medical branch of Siemens-Reiniger in Erlangen.[12] Their experiments

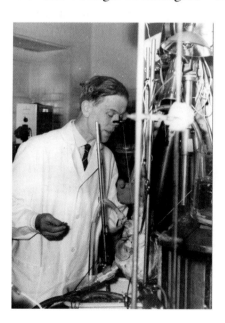

Fig. 9.2. Inge Edler with the experimental set-up for studying ultrasonic echoes in the heart. (Courtesy of the South Swedish Society for the History of Medicine.)

were carried out *in vitro* and *in vivo*. Much of this early testing used calf hearts, with movements obtained by connecting the heart to a fluid pump. Indeed, some of this work was carried out in the kitchen of an unused medical ward before being tested on hospital patients.[8]

Initially Edler and Hertz developed an A-mode (amplitude-mode) device, a technique that plotted the returning echoes as a function of the depth relative to the transducer, for echocardiographic studies, but soon realised that this display did not yield practical information for cardiac diagnosis; it was only able to detect the depth at which the acoustic impedance difference was originating and the amplitude of the reflected sound. The machine was also not able to record movement and a recording device was therefore needed.[7]

In 1953, Hertz and Edler received a new Siemens machine with the addition of a photographic TM-mode (time-motion-mode) recorder. This recorder allowed simultaneous recording of the electrocardiogram (ECG), and the results were therefore called ultrasonic cardiograms (UCG)[12] (Fig. 9.3). The echoes were from the posterior wall of the left ventricle and from what was then assumed to be the left atrium. On 29 October 1953, the first ultrasound cardiogram was created. This work of Edler and Hertz was published in the *Proceedings*

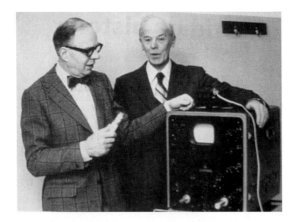

Fig. 9.3. Carl Hellmuth Hertz and Inge Edler with the ultrasound reflectoscope that was used for the recordings of the first echocardiograms. (Courtesy of the South Swedish Society for the History of Medicine.)

of the Royal Physiological Society in Lund in 1954 and entitled 'The Use of the Ultrasonic Reflectoscope for Continuous Movements of the Heart Wall'.[8]

The contribution of engineering, in particular the development of viewing monitors, was extremely valuable to the development of ultrasound. In 1956, the TM method of viewing heart wall motion directly onto the face of a cathode ray tube came into general use.[12] Siemens built a barium titanate transducer in 1958 especially for Edler and Hertz,[12] allowing them to record normal mitral valve motion as well as to observe other structures in the heart.[5] This allowed the observation of a consistent pattern of recordings in normal patients that differed from the recordings from patients who had mitral valve disease.[13] Edler and Hertz subsequently used ultrasound to detect fluid in the pericardium, blood clots and atrial myxomas.[2]

In 1959, the duo revealed that the second echo that they had identified on the ultrasonic cardiogram was actually from the anterior leaflet of the mitral valve. Edler realised this by carrying out experiments on human autopsies and on dying patients. 'Edler marked the location and angle of the ultrasonic beam on a patient, and once the patient had died, stuck an ice pick in the direction of the beam. On the subsequent post-mortem he discovered the ice pick in the anterior mitral valve leaflet.'[4] This was the cornerstone in pre-operative mitral value surgery evaluation[7] and was shown on a pre-recorded film at the Third European Congress of Cardiology in Rome in 1960. Edler was the first to demonstrate the motion of the anterior leaflet of the mitral valve and the effect of mitral stenosis.[11] It had been difficult for Edler and Hertz to reach the correct conclusion about the source of their echoes earlier because of a lack of knowledge of the ultrasonic properties of the different tissues of the heart.[12]

Edler and Hertz performed their work in adults with co-workers at the University Hospital in Lund. Similar work in paediatrics was subsequently performed by Nils-Rune Lundström. The transducers used at that time were made out of quartz, with a sensitivity 100 times less than modern ceramic transducers.[6]

Many papers were published in Scandinavian journals, and echocardiography was rapidly becoming routine practice in Lund. Despite these advances, there were difficulties in getting other clinicians to apply the method even within the Scandinavian countries.[8] Although there were many visitors to their laboratory in Lund during the 1950s the ultrasound method still did not become widely accepted. Hertz forwarded Edler's 1961 publication, 'The use of ultrasound as a diagnostic aid, and its effects on biological tissues'[14] to his former colleagues in the US and subsequently in 1962 Edler was invited to present their work at a conference in Ubana, Illinois.[12] This finally ignited enthusiasm and others started using this new ultrasound technique and sharing ideas.[10] This was when the term echocardiography was first used, coined by the American Society of Ultrasound in Medicine.[10]

As interest in the use of ultrasound grew, Edler and Hertz made several visits to cardiologists and to electronics factories to develop and improve ultrasound techniques. The engineering industry likewise became interested in this new ultrasound development, which encouraged improvements to the existing reflectoscopes to meet the demands made by echocardiography.[12]

Although Edler and Hertz worked together they did not publish a great deal as co-authors. Following the medical community's acceptance of the practice of echocardiography, both Edler and Hertz gradually branched out into differing aspects of this field.

Hertz and his co-workers concentrated on creating two-dimensional (2D) echocardiography. Hertz gradually improved this method by using mechanical mirror systems to enable the images to be presented in real time, conducting this work in the Department of Technology at Lund University in 1967.[6] Although this breakthrough was achieved primarily by Hertz and his team, Edler remained in close co-operation. However, the Swedish Board of Technological Development did not feel that the project had had enough medical and commercial development and this aspect of Hertz's work was further developed outside Sweden.[8]

At the beginning of the 1960s, Edler (in collaboration with Nils-Rune Lundström) used ultrasound Doppler equipment to identify intracardiac blood flow, soon after clinical equipment for estimating blood flow in superficial arteries became available. As Edler was experienced in cardiac auscultation and phonocardiography he was convinced that he could hear blood flow,[6] and is quoted as saying, 'these results were convincing and the results of Doppler signals from the inside of the heart generated by blood flow were recorded'.[6] This work on isolated heart preparations as well as in patients was presented at the first World Congress on Ultrasound Diagnosis in Vienna in 1969 by Edler and Lundström. This presentation included the first 40 intracardiac Doppler recordings in patients with mitral and aortic valve incompetence.[6] This was the last occasion that Edler published his research, and he retired in 1977.[4]

Although 2D echocardiography and Doppler developed simultaneously, 2D echo was perceived as the 'easier' technique and acceptable by cardiologists who brought this method into regular clinical use several years before Doppler.[8] The Doppler method first used has now evolved and advanced to become the colour Doppler technique that is in routine use today and has promoted major changes in the ultrasound diagnosis and management of cardiac disease.

It was in the 1970s that ultrasound became widely accepted[3] leading to the very first international congress on echocardiography in 1980.

M-mode (motion-mode) curves were, and still are, produced by a series of ultrasound pulses being emitted sequentially to determine the velocity of a structure relative to the transducer. In the 1980s, Hertz also focused on the development of ink-jet technology that could be used to record echocardiographic M-mode curves. Hertz invented a method to electrically control tiny ink droplets, the forerunner of the now widely used ink jet colour printer.[9]

From these early and important developments in cardiology, where Edler and Hertz made enormous contributions, many other workers could see the potential of ultrasound and strove to apply the technology to their group of patients. Others were working at the same time as Edler and Hertz, coming to the same appreciation of the utility and flexibility of ultrasound in the context of patient

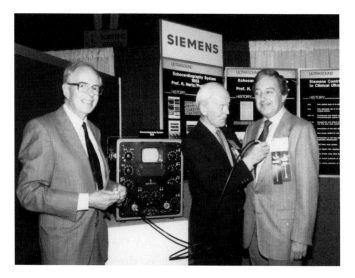

Fig. 9.4.   Carl Hellmuth Hertz and Inge Edler in a Siemens booth, examining the heart of Barry Goldberg of Thomas Jefferson Hospital, Philadelphia. (Courtesy of the South Swedish Society for the History of Medicine.)

management; the technique was adopted by physicians and scientists across the globe (Fig. 9.4).

9.5   Other Applications of Ultrasound

9.5.1   *Paediatrics*

Ultrasound, as an entirely non-invasive technique, was appreciated as a way of imaging children by Nils-Rune Lundström, a paediatric cardiologist in Lund. Lundström's initial acceptance of the use of ultrasound echocardiography followed his encounter with a patient with cor triatriatum, a condition with an obstructing membrane in the left atrium. Ultrasound examination pre- and post-surgery convinced him of the value of echocardiography in paediatrics. Lundström's work was presented at the World Congress on Ultrasound Diagnosis in Vienna in 1969 where he showed several congenital heart defects such as Ebstein's anomaly, congenital mitral stenosis, hypoplastic left heart syndrome, cor triatriatum and membranous subaortic stenosis.

Lundström then went on to publish several other articles including a series in *Acta Paediatrica Scandanavica* on normal values of various intracardiac measurements in paediatrics and the clinical applications of echocardiography in the paediatric population.[8]

9.5.2 Echoencephalography

In the late 1930s and early 1940s, Karl Theo Dussik investigated the use of ultrasound in tumour detection within the brain.[11] Dussik was a neurologist at the University of Vienna who is regarded as the first physician to have used ultrasound in clinical diagnosis.[1] He mounted transducers on either side of the head and measured ultrasound transmission profiles, 'hyperphonograms', and claimed to be able to detect tumours. Subsequently he worked with neurosurgeons and engineers at the Massachusetts Institute of Technology (MIT) attempting to detect all types of intracranial pathology. The work was criticised due to the attenuation of the beam by the skull and the images were deemed to be artefacts; the project was terminated and no further work was done by Dussik or his colleagues at MIT.

Lars Leksell was a Swedish neurosurgeon working in Lund, where he developed the concept of radiosurgery and the gamma knife, a method where gamma radiation was directed to a target point in the patient's brain.[15] Leksell utilised an ultrasound machine that he had borrowed from Edler and Hertz, which was used to examine children with thin skull bones. Using the A-mode method he evaluated the distance from the scalp to the calcified pineal gland. Leksell commented that 'lateral displacement of the calcified pineal body in the echoencephalogram is a valuable diagnostic sign of an expanding intracranial lesion', e.g. haemorrhage or tumour. Echoencephalography was first successfully undertaken on 16 December 1953 and therefore developed as a spin-off of echocardiography and the pioneering work of Edler and Hertz.[15]

9.5.3 Ultrasound in obstetrics and gynaecology

The pioneering work on the use of ultrasound in obstetrics and gynaecology was undertaken by Ian Donald, a Glaswegian obstetrician.

Donald was described as 'no backroom boffin, but a full-blown flamboyant consultant at the sharp edge of one of medicine's most acute specialities'.[1] In 1954, Donald travelled to a nuclear plant where ultrasound was used for metal flaw detection. He saw its diagnostic potential and subsequently borrowed an A-mode unit from the Royal Marsden Hospital, London. Donald carried out several experiments on pelvic masses that had been surgically removed and discovered that he was able to image ovarian cysts, ascites and hydramnios in his patients.[11]

Donald, together with his colleagues, Tom Brown (an engineer) and John MacVicar (Donald's Registrar), created a contact scanner that was fixed to an examination table and mounted over the patient. Crude pictures were obtained as the transducer was moved manually over the patient. Donald and his colleagues were able to identify a large operable ovarian cyst in a woman who had been given the diagnosis of inoperable stomach cancer.[1] Donald's work was published in the *Lancet* in 1958 and entitled 'Investigation of Abdominal Masses by Pulsed Ultrasound',[16] encouraging the medical profession to take more notice of the possibilities offered by ultrasound. The latter was consequently used in early pregnancy to assess positioning of the foetus, twins and malformations. Donald was able to show that ultrasound was not harmful to the foetus and was the first to measure biparietal diameters as an index of foetal growth in 1962.

At the same time, Joseph Holmes and colleagues at the University of Colorado created a compound contact scanner that was moved along an overhead track and across the patient's abdomen. They were the first to demonstrate an echo pattern from the placenta and this scanner and their work, together with Donald's, removed much of the scepticism about the use of ultrasound in obstetrics.[11]

9.5.4 *Doppler ultrasound*

In 1842, Christian Andreas Doppler, Austrian mathematician and physicist, was the first to 'analyze the effect of motion of the observer relative to the source of a wave on the perceived wave frequency, known as Doppler Effect'.[4]

Ultrasound Doppler technique for vascular applications was developed in 1956 by Shigeo Satomura of Osaka University in Japan. Satomura's results were interpreted as caused by movements of the heart muscle and a valve rather than blood flow, but at the time were thought to be of insignificant cardiological interest.[6] The development of Doppler echocardiography paralleled Edler and Hertz's development of M-mode and 2D echocardiography.

From 1958 onwards Donald Baker and Robert Rushmer, American investigators, incorporated Doppler techniques into cardiac ultrasound machines and published the first transcutaneous vascular spectral flow signals.[1,4] This was a breakthrough, as it now established a way to quantify pressure drops across valvular stenoses.[4]

In 1985, in Tokyo, Japan, Chihiro Kasai and his co-workers, who were a group of bioengineers and cardiologists, introduced a colour Doppler flow-mapping system that combined Doppler flow with B-mode[3] (brightness-mode) so that blood flow could be visualised non-invasively; the real-time colour flow imaging that is used today that allows us to use a linear array transducer to obtain 2D images of the body (Fig. 9.5).

9.5.5 *Contrast enhanced ultrasound*

Raymond Gramiak and Pravin Shah are considered to be pioneers in the use of contrast agents in ultrasound. In 1969 they used 'intracardiac injection of substances that produce echoes at the site of injection as well as downstream in the flow pattern and permit identification of the heart cavities'.[17] Initially they used saline but found improved results with agitated saline and then indocyanine green dye, normal saline and 5% dextrose to improve visualisation of cardiac chambers.[18]

The need for contrast in ultrasound developed when researchers realised that distinguishing normal from abnormal tissues on greyscale images was difficult when they had similar tissue properties. Contrast agents enhance backscatter and have therefore been used to enhance the echogenicity of blood and improve the Doppler signal or increase the contrast between normal and abnormal tissues.[19]

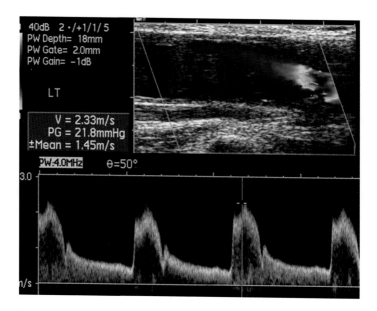

Fig. 9.5.   A modern-day image of the carotid artery incorporating B-mode, colour Doppler and spectral Doppler technique, displayed in real time and simultaneously. The image demonstrates a carotid artery that is 6 mm in diameter, filled with thrombus, with a 'jet' of colour representing a stenosis, with the velocity measured with Doppler techniques.

Marvin C. Ziskin proved in 1972 that the reflectivity of contrast was due to the presence of microbubbles of gas which 'went back into solution over time'.[19] Microbubbles are non-toxic encapsulated gas bubbles that resonate at various frequencies. It has been shown that the safety of microbubbles is comparable to the contrast agents used in computed tomography or magnetic resonance imaging.[20]

In the future we may find that microbubbles may be used to aid drug delivery to a specific site within the body. 'Ultrasound can potentiate drug delivery by creating transient non-lethal perforations in cell membranes to aid ingress of large molecules and particles into cells (sonoporation).'[20]

9.5.6 Elastography

Elastography is the technique that utilises the properties of tissue displacement to delineate lesions and the principles of palpation to assess the mechanical properties of tissues.[3] The aim of shear wave elastography is to produce images that describe the spatial and temporal variations in tissue viscoelasticity.[21]

It was developed in France and Belgium in the 1970s for assessing tissue stiffness by observing M-mode features during palpation. Similar work was then done in the 1980s by European and Japanese researchers but with B-mode. The first elastography image was made and shown at the annual conference of The American Institute for Ultrasound in Medicine (1988).[21] Elastography is used to distinguish benign from malignant lesions, to identify hepatic fibrosis and in breast imaging. Further research into its applications is continuing.

9.6 The Impact of these Discoveries on Medical Science

The development of echocardiography has revolutionised clinical practice and ultrasound is the second most commonly utilised diagnostic imaging modality.[3] It is non-ionising, cheap, portable, has resolution in the millimetre range and allows for blood flow information from Doppler techniques.[3]

It has been almost 60 years since Edler and Hertz introduced echocardiography. The development occurred despite the lack of high-speed electronics, fast computers and advanced ultrasonic transducers. It has not only advanced the clinical use of ultrasound but promoted further development of information technology and electronics.[6]

The development of echocardiography was successful not only because of the brilliant minds and dedication of Edler and Hertz but also because of their close collaboration, despite coming from different fields. Edler and Hertz were able to learn from one another and share ideas, their synergism resulting in a discovery that has now changed medicine. Hertz himself recognised that further work needed to be conducted following their initial results and said that 'the first lucky strike of discovery will not give lasting results if it is not followed up by such a conscientious and considerable effort by many other workers'.[12]

References

1. Woo J, 2002. *History of Ultrasound in Obstetrics and Gynaecology.* Available online at: http://www.ob-ultrasound.net/history.html (Accessed: 3 November 2012).
2. Nilson J, Westling N. Ultrasound in Lund — three world premieres. *Clinical Physiology and Functional Imaging* 2004; 24: 137–140.
3. Shung KK. Diagnostic Ultrasound: Past, Present, and Future. *Journal of Medical and Biological Engineering* 2010; 31: 371–374.
4. Gowda RM, Khan IA, Vasavada BC *et al.* History of the evolution of echocardiography. *International Journal of Cardiology* 2004; 97: 1–6.
5. Thomas AMK, Banerjee AK, Busch U. *Classic Papers in Modern Diagnostic Radiology.* Berlin: Springer; 2005.
6. Holmer N, Lindström K, Lundström N *et al.* In Memoriam: Inge Edler — the father of echocardiography. *European Journal of Ultrasound* 2001; 13: 179–182.
7. Westling H. Ultrasound in Lund — three world premieres. In: Eklöf B, Lindström K, Persson S (eds), *Ultrasound in Clinical Diagnosis — From Pioneering Developments in Lund to Global Application in Medicine.* Oxford: Oxford University Press; 2012: pp. 1–7.
8. Persson S, Eskilsson J, Lundström N. The development of echocardiology in Sweden. In: Eklöf B, Lindström K, Persson S (eds), *Ultrasound in Clinical Diagnosis — From Pioneering Developments in Lund to Global Application in Medicine.* Oxford: Oxford University Press; 2012: pp. 8–20.
9. Lindström K. Carl Hellmuth Hertz — A Tribute. *Ultrasound in Medicine and Biology* 1991; 17: 421–424.
10. Fraser AG. Inge Edler and the Origins of Clinical Echocardiography. *Eur J Echocardiography* 2001; 2: 3–5.
11. Hendee WR. Cross sectional medical imaging: A History. *Radiographics* 1989; 9: 1155–1180.
12. Hertz CH. The interaction of physicians, physicists and industry in the development of echocardiography. *Ultrasound in Medicine and Biology* 1973; 1: 3–11.
13. Segal BL. Symposium on Echocardiography (Diagnostic Ultrasound). *The American Journal of Cardiology* 1967; 19: 1–5.

14. Edler I. The use of ultrasound as a diagnostic aid, and its effects on biological tissues. *Acta Med Scand Suppl* 1961; 370: 7–65.

15. Salford LG. The development of echoencephalography in Sweden. In: Eklöf B, Lindström K, Persson S (eds), *Ultrasound in Clinical Diagnosis — From Pioneering Developments in Lund to Global Application in Medicine.* Oxford: Oxford University Press; 2012: pp. 43–49.

16. Donald I. MacVicar, J, Brown TG. Investigation of abdominal masses by pulsed ultrasound. *Lancet* 1958; 1: 1188–1195.

17. Gramiak R, Shah PM, Kramer DH. Ultrasound cardiography: Contrast Studies in Anatomy and Function. *Radiology* 1969; 92: 939–948.

18. Sorrell VL, Kumar S. Doppler Contrast Echocardiography. In: Fleming RM (ed.), *Establishing Better Standards of Care in Doppler Echocardiography, Computed Tomography and Nuclear Cardiology.* Shanghai: In Tech; 2011, 135–146.

19. Goldberg BB, Liu J, Forsberg F. Ultrasound contrast agents. *Ultrasound in Medicine and Biology* 1994; 20: 319–333.

20. Blomley MJ, Cooke JC, Unger EC *et al.* Microbubble contrast agents: A new era in ultrasound. *BMJ* 2001; 322: 1222–1225.

21. Bamber JC. Comment on new technology — ultrasound elastography. *Ultraschall Med* 2008; 29: 319–320.

22. Eklöf B, Lindström K, Persson S. Preface. In: Eklöf B, Lindström K, Persson S (eds), *Ultrasound in Clinical Diagnosis — From Pioneering Developments in Lund to Global Application in Medicine.* Oxford: Oxford University Press; 2012: pp. ix–xi.

Appendix A[22]

Inge Edler — National and International Distinctions:

1971   Honorary member of the American Ultrasound Association
1974   Honorary member of the German Ultrasound Association
1977   Albert Lasker Clinical Medical Research Award
1978   Honorary member of the Swedish Ultrasound Association
1979   Honorary member of the Yugoslavian Ultrasound Association
1983   Rotterdam Echocardiography Award
1984   Award for scientific work of extraordinary significance from the Royal Physiographic Society of Lund
1987   Honorary member of the Swedish Society of Cardiology
1988   Aachen and Munich Prize for Technology and Applied Sciences

History of Medical Ultrasound Pioneer Award from the American Institute of Ultrasound in Medicine, the World Federation of Ultrasound in Medicine and Biology and the Medical Sciences Division of the National Museum of American History, Smithsonian Institution (Washington)
1991   Eric K. Fernström's Great Nordic Prize
Honorary member of the American College of Cardiology
2000   Chosen as 'The Swedish Cardiologist of the 20th Century' by the Swedish Cardiology Society

Modified from: Persson S., Eskilsson J. and Lundström N. The development of echocardiology in Sweden. In: Eklöf B, Lindström K, Persson S (eds). *Ultrasound in Clinical Diagnosis — From Pioneering Developments in Lund to Global Application in Medicine.* Oxford: Oxford University Press; 2012.

Appendix B[9]

Hellmuth Hertz — National and International Distinctions:

1966 Ebeling Prize from Swedish Society of Medical Sciences
1971 Honorary Fellow of American Institute of Ultrasound in Medicine
1977 Albert Lasker Clinical Medical Research Award
1978 Honorary doctor's degree from medical faculty Lund University
1983 Rotterdam Echocardiography Award
1984 Award for scientific work of extraordinary significance from the Royal Physiographic Society of Lund
1986 Albert Rose Electronic Imager of the Year Award for work on ink-jet technology
1988 Johann Gutenberg Prize from the Society of Information Display, US
Lecturer of the Year Award of the Society for Imaging Science and Technology (SPSE)
Aachen and Munich Prize for Technology and Applied Sciences
The Grand Inventor Prize from the Swedish Board for Technical Developments (STU) for important technical innovations
History of Medical Ultrasound Pioneer Award from the American Institute of Ultrasound in Medicine, the World Federation of Ultrasound in Medicine and Biology and the Medical Sciences Division of the National Museum of American History, Smithsonian Institution (Washington)
Upon retirement he became the first Emeritus member of the editorial board of *Ultrasound in Medicine and Biology*

Modified from: Lindström K. Carl Hellmuth Hertz — A Tribute. *Ultrasound in Medicine and Biology* 1991; **17**(5): 421–424.

Chapter 10

CYRIL CLARKE, RONALD FINN, JOHN GORMAN, VINCENT FREDA AND WILLIAM POLLACK: THE PREVENTION OF Rh HAEMOLYTIC DISEASE OF THE NEWBORN

David J. Weatherall

10.1 Introduction

There is no doubt that the research that led to the successful prevention of Rhesus (Rh) haemolytic disease of the newborn in the 1960s, carried out quite independently by teams in Liverpool and New York, was one of the major successes of public health and preventative medicine in the second half of the 20th century. But although the importance of this work was reflected by the presentation of the prestigious Lasker Award to two members of the Liverpool team and three members of the New York team in 1980, this extremely important advance in preventative medicine was never recognised by the Nobel Prize Committee.

The story of the discovery of the Rh blood group system and its complexity, how Rh incompatibility between a mother and fetus leads to haemolytic disease of the newborn, and the evolution of approaches to symptomatic management of this condition are discussed in detail elsewhere.[1,2] Here, we will examine the backgrounds and work of the Liverpool and New York teams in an attempt to understand why this work, given its seminal medical importance, was never recognised by the Nobel Prize Committee.

10.2 The Work of the Liverpool Team

10.2.1 *Background*

The leader of the Liverpool team was the remarkable physician Cyril Astley Clarke (Fig. 10.1). There have been several extensive accounts of his life and work,[3,4] including two informal autobiographical pieces that he wrote in his 88th year.[5,6] He was born in Leicester on 22 August 1902. His father was a physician at Leicester Royal Infirmary and one of the first in the UK to use diagnostic X-rays. After his school years he was admitted to Caius College, Cambridge, to read Natural Sciences. In 1929, he left Cambridge and entered Guy's Hospital Medical School where he qualified in medicine in 1936. For the next three years he worked in a life insurance practice in London, during which time he also obtained the MRCP qualification and an MD from Cambridge. After service in the navy during World War II, and a short period as a Registrar at Queen Elizabeth Hospital, Birmingham, he was appointed as a Consultant Physician to the

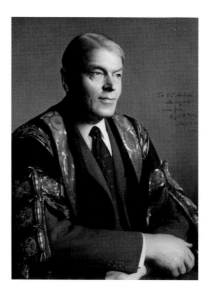

Fig. 10.1. Sir Cyril Clarke on the occasion of his appointment as President of the Royal College of Physicians, London after his retirement in 1972. (A signed photograph given to the author.)

David Lewis Northern Hospital in Liverpool in 1946. Here, as well as general medicine, he developed a special interest in asthma and also evolved a flourishing private practice.

Since his schooldays, Clarke had been fascinated by butterflies and despite his busy clinical career in Liverpool he started to study the swallowtail butterfly, *Papilio machaon*. Through this work, in 1952 he met Philip Sheppard, a geneticist working in Oxford who later moved to Liverpool to become its first Professor of Genetics in 1963. The extensive work that Clarke and Sheppard carried out on the evolution of mimicry in butterflies is described elsewhere[3] and is remembered through the Clarke–Sheppard–Gill collection of butterflies in the Natural History Museum.

During this period, as Clarke recalls in one of his memoirs,[5] he asked Philip Sheppard how he could apply his increasing knowledge of genetics to medicine. Sheppard's advice was through the study of blood groups and, as Clarke wrote later, 'blood groups it was'. After early studies on the relationship between blood groups and duodenal ulcer he started to build up a young team of clinicians working on various aspects of blood groups and disease.[7]

10.2.2 Beginnings of work on Rh haemolytic disease of the newborn

In his later writings about the Liverpool research programme at this time,[5,6] Clarke suggested that the study of the Rhesus blood group system was a natural extension of his work on butterflies. He likened the closely linked Rh loci on chromosome 1 to similar families of linked genes responsible for mimicry in swallowtail butterflies. Although this may be a rather generous stretch of the imagination, at about this time he decided to look again at some previously reported observations on the relationship between maternal ABO blood groups and Rhesus sensitisation.

In the 1950s, the usual pathway for training young consultant physicians was for them to obtain the MD degree from a research-based thesis followed by a spell in the United States. In 1957, Clarke was approached by a young Senior House Officer, Ronald Finn

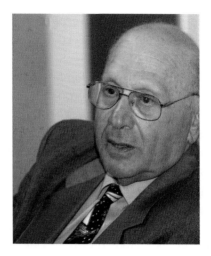

Fig. 10.2.   Ronald Finn. A photograph taken at the Wellcome Witness to 20th Century Medicine Meeting on The Rhesus Factor and Disease Prevention in 2004. (By kind permission of the Wellcome Trust Photographic Library.)

(Fig. 10.2), a University of Liverpool graduate who was training in general medicine and nephrology, with a request for a project that would lead to an MD qualification. Clarke suggested that it might be interesting to re-examine an earlier observation that fetomaternal ABO blood group incompatibility protects against the development of Rhesus haemolytic disease. Finn took on this project and soon confirmed these earlier findings. While he was completing these studies two extremely important papers appeared. First, Kleihauer and his team in Germany showed that it is possible to identify fetal red cells in adult blood by a simple acid-elution slide-staining technique.[8] Two years later, in 1959, Zipursky and his group in Toronto showed that it is possible to identify fetal red cells in the maternal circulation by using this approach.[9] In completing his thesis work Finn used the acid-elution technique to analyse the frequency of cross-placental passage of fetal cells in pregnancy and found that they are present in the blood of nearly 12% of women in the early post-partum period. Even more importantly, he also noted an association between the development of Rh antibodies and the size of these fetal bleeds into the maternal circulation. Furthermore, fetal cells were never found in maternal blood when the fetus and mother were ABO incompatible.[10] This suggested that circulating Rh-positive fetal cells in an Rh-negative mother might be similarly selectively destroyed or inactivated by the administration of a strong Rh antibody, anti-D for example.[2] In short, this might be an approach to preventing Rh sensitisation of the mother.

It is interesting to ask, or at least speculate, on which member of the Liverpool team actually was first to suggest the administration of anti-RhD for the prevention of haemolytic disease of the newborn. Several times Clarke suggested that it was his wife, Feo, who woke up in the middle of the night after a dream and shouted, 'Give them anti-D!'[11] Although this sounds highly unlikely, it is important to point out that although Feo Clarke had no formal training in any branch of medicine or science, she was an extremely intelligent person who was absolutely critical in Clarke's work, always helping him to write and re-write his scientific papers. However, the first published suggestion regarding the use of anti-D appeared in a short account of a paper that Finn gave at a Symposium entitled 'The Role of Inheritance in Common Diseases' that was held at the Liverpool Medical Institution on 18 February 1960, an abstract of which was later published in the *Lancet*.[12] This question was further discussed at the Wellcome Witness Seminar on the Rhesus Factor and Disease Prevention in 2004.[2] Finn suggested that, because Feo Clarke edited and classified all the published work from Clarke's group at the time, and that it was he who had organised and run the Symposium, she might have come across this abstract and mentioned its contents to Clarke, though Finn was far from sure whether she had actually suggested this approach. In short, although we will never know who first suggested this concept it seems likely that it was either Clarke or Finn!

10.2.3 *A successful outcome to the hypothesis*

By the early 1960s, a small team had been built up around Clarke and Finn which set out to test the idea that it might be possible to prevent haemolytic disease of the newborn by inactivating or destroying the cells from Rh-positive fetuses that had crossed the placenta into the circulation of Rh-negative mothers.[2] It included Philip Sheppard, Clarke's long-term colleague; Richard McConnell, a general physician and gastroenterologist who had also worked with Clarke on most of his projects over the years; John Woodrow, a general physician and rheumatologist with a major interest in immunology who had carried out some of the classical studies relating Type 1 diabetes to the human leucocyte antigen (HLA) system; and Shona Towers, an obstetrician. All the laboratory work was carried out by a senior technician, Bill Donohoe, and the team was helped on the blood transfusion aspects of their programmes by Dermot Lehane of the Liverpool Blood Transfusion Service.

But how to test the hypothesis? Clarke wrote later: 'We could not test it on women of child-bearing age so we started experiments on volunteer Rh-negative male policemen who were extremely co-operative and who, when warned that the work might produce all sorts of dire consequences, including leukaemia, replied that they trusted their doctors! They believed they might really be doing some good and, mercifully, there were no ethical committees in those days.'[5]

Early experiments in these male volunteers, which analysed the clearance of Rh-positive cells by administering complete (19S) anti-D serum, suggested that immunisation was enhanced rather than prevented. Following the suggestion of Ruth Sanger, the studies were repeated using incomplete (7S) anti-D and the results seemed to be more promising. When the team obtained some Ortho anti-D-gamma globulin, this was found to be even more effective than the serum that they had been using. Further work, this time on female volunteers, suggested that they were moving in the right direction, while at the same time they found that consequential analysis of the blood of pregnant women indicated that the main trans-placental passage of fetal cells takes place either just before or after delivery. Both Finn and Woodrow subsequently carried out a similar series of experiments while Research Fellows at Johns Hopkins Hospital, Baltimore, with the help of the haematologist Julius Krevans; in this case the male volunteers were prisoners in the Baltimore Penitentiary, rather than policemen. Following a series of seminal papers describing these early studies, the Liverpool team felt that they were now ready to perform a major clinical trial for the prevention of Rhesus sensitisation in pregnant women.[10,13,14]

The first trial was carried out jointly between several centres in England and in Baltimore. The results showed that the injection of anti-D given shortly after delivery resulted in no case of Rh sensitisation in 78 treated women; 19 of a similar number of controls showed sensitisation.[15] In 1971, the authors published a follow-up study of the high-risk women who had been treated and found that the failure rate was only 2.3% whereas 30.7% of the controls were sensitised after their second Rh-positive pregnancy.[16] It is likely that the high sensitisation rate in these studies reflected the fact that the women in the study were at high risk of sensitisation as judged by the number of fetal cells found in their circulation after delivery of their first baby. Indeed, it was Philip Sheppard who insisted that the first trial should recruit only women at high risk of sensitisation.

After this remarkable success story we must briefly leave the Liverpool scene and find out what was happening in New York at this time.

10.3 The Work of the New York Team in Prevention of Rh Haemolytic Disease of the Newborn

10.3.1 *Background*

The work of the New York team in this field is recounted in two extensive monographs,[17,18] one of which[18] has a foreword giving insight into its nature by James D. Watson, the co-discoverer of the structure of DNA. From these accounts of the studies in New York it is absolutely clear that they were carried out quite independently and that the scientists involved only heard about what was happening in Liverpool when their studies were well advanced.

The research in New York was carried out by three clinical scientists, John Gorman, Vincent Freda and William Pollock. John Gorman (Fig. 10.3), who was 28 years old when the programme started and nearing the end of his pathology training in the Blood

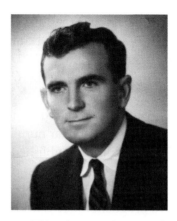

Fig. 10.3. John Gorman. This photograph was taken during the period of Gorman's work on Rhesus prevention and was kindly provided by him.

Bank at the Columbia-Presbyterian Medical Center in New York, was born in Australia and obtained his medical degree at the University of Melbourne. After a year's internship he moved to the United States in 1955 and began a period of training in pathology at Columbia-Presbyterian. Probably because of the strong influence of his teachers in Australia he had a major interest in immunology and genetics and the beginnings of a particular research interest in immunohaematology. It was undoubtedly this background which stimulated his interest in Rhesus haemolytic disease.

Vincent Freda was born in New Haven, Connecticut, and received his medical training at New York University Medical Center where he became interested in obstetrics. After military service he returned to New York University for the early part of his obstetric training, which he completed at the Columbia-Presbyterian Medical Center. Because of his growing interest in immunohaematology and Rhesus disease he arranged to spend the fifth year of his residency training working with Alexander Wiener, the co-discoverer of the Rhesus blood group system, at New York University. It was during this time that he became fascinated with the possibility of research into the prevention of Rh haemolytic disease. On returning to Columbia-Presbyterian he established a serology laboratory and, later, through an attachment to the Blood Bank, he first encountered John Gorman.

The third member of the team, William Pollack, was an Englishman who had trained at Imperial College in London, where he obtained a Bachelor's Degree in chemistry and physics and, later, he obtained a Master's Degree in biochemistry and physiology at St George's Hospital Medical School, London. He then moved to the US where he obtained his PhD in immunochemistry from Rutgers University in New Jersey. In the mid-1950s, he moved to Canada and became Chief of the clinical laboratories at a hospital in Vancouver, where he produced several valuable diagnostic agents for use in blood testing. This work led to an offer of a post in Ortho to which he moved in 1956. Part of his agreement with the pharmaceutical company was that he should receive both time and suitable equipment and laboratory space to conduct research of his own choice. By the time he first met John Gorman he was already involved in a programme of study of the immunochemistry of the Rh antigen-antibody response.

10.3.2 *Trials of antibody-induced immunodepression*

As discussed in Gorman's description of the New York programme[17] it was preceded by an extensive review of the early literature on antibody-induced immunodepression (AID). In 1960, the New York team set out a comprehensive proposal to develop AID into a practical public health measure to prevent Rh haemolytic disease of the newborn. In essence they decided to develop Rh immune globulin, an injectable concentrate of anti-Rh which was shown to render Rh-negative mothers refractory to immunisation by Rh-positive blood. Their programme evolved along similar lines to that in Liverpool, first by the study of protection in Rh-negative males and later to clinical trials in Rh-negative mothers.

In contrast to the Liverpool team, the New York team chose from the beginning to use as its immunosuppressant intra-muscular gamma globulin fractionated from plasma containing anti-Rh. Also, unlike the Liverpool group which carried out its early experiments on male volunteers using policemen, the early work on Rh-negative male volunteers in New York was carried out on volunteer prisoners at Sing Sing Prison. After two years of trials at Sing Sing it was clear that Rh immunoglobulin in adequate dosage provided 100% protection against sensitisation by a level of antigenic stimulus which was much greater than that of the usual Rh-positive pregnancy and, even more importantly, without any unwanted side effects.[19] These extremely promising findings were followed by a clinical trial at Columbia University College of Physicians and Surgeons which included 346 treated and 151 control women. There were no sensitised women in the treated group either six months post-partum or at the next delivery.[19,20] Shortly after this trial began, and after two other smaller trials in the US, it became apparent to Ortho that an expanded study would be needed and the programme was extended to 43 centres in the US, Canada, Australia, Ireland and Scotland. The data from this larger trial clearly established the effectiveness of this approach to prevention of Rh haemolytic disease. The final figures together with appropriate references are summarised in Gorman's monograph.[17] In short, in the major international study only six of over 3,000 treated patients were sensitised at six months post-partum, whereas 102 out of over 1,000 controls were sensitised.

Further trials were carried out based on the Liverpool and New York proposals, notably in West Germany[21] and St. Louis,[22,23] and by the early 1970s it was absolutely clear that, although a great deal more organisational work would be required, together with investigation of the production and pharmacology of Rh immune globulin, it was now certain that it would be possible to prevent the majority of cases of Rh haemolytic disease of the newborn — a truly remarkable achievement. There is a valuable collection of selected papers and extracts edited by Clarke which cover both the earlier period of this research and some of the international problems in establishing the prevention of Rh haemolytic disease in clinical practice.[24] And some of Woodrow's early and later thoughts about the possible immune mechanisms involved in the success of the anti-D approach are also available.[3,25]

The current approach to the prevention of Rh haemolytic disease is described in detail elsewhere[26] and will only be outlined here. All pregnant women who are Rh negative receive a standard dose of anti-D within 72 hours of delivery. The Kleihauer test is carried out and if there is an unusually large fetomaternal haemorrhage a supplementary dose of anti-D is given immediately and a repeat test for fetal cells and free anti-D is carried out on the mother 48 hours after the initial anti-D injection. A further supplementary dose of anti-D may be required if there is no free anti-D detectable in the mother or if fetal cells are still present. Anti-D is also given in abortion, ectopic pregnancy, after amniocentesis and a variety of other conditions. In the UK every year 80,000 RhD-negative women have an RhD-positive infant and despite national guidelines sensitisation still occurs, mainly due to non-compliance with these guidelines.

10.4 A Brief Summary of the Backgrounds and Roads to Success of the Liverpool and New York Teams

One of the most remarkable features of this extraordinary success story is undoubtedly the completely different background of those who comprised the teams that were involved. Apart from Clarke's knowledge of genetics gained through his hobby of studying the inheritance of mimicry in butterflies and his support by Sheppard, who was a first class geneticist by training, none of the team had any background in haematology or blood group serology. Indeed, in Liverpool at that time any form of specialisation was frowned upon, largely through the influence of the Professor of Medicine, Lord Cohen, whose view was that a specialist was one who knew everything about the subject except its relative importance! Furthermore, none of the early members of the team had any background or training in immunology although this deficiency was corrected to some degree when Woodrow joined them. But in a later discussion about the work of the Liverpool team,[2] Finn and Woodrow made it quite clear that they felt that they were considered to be a group of amateurs by those who ran the blood transfusion service or who were experts in the field of blood group serology in the UK! And serendipity also played a role in the Liverpool programme. There is little doubt that the papers that appeared on how to identify fetal red cells while Finn was carrying out his initial studies on the protective effect of ABO incompatibility on Rh sensitisation undoubtedly played a major role in moving the work forward and in raising the possibility of an approach to prevention of Rh haemolytic disease. Another remarkable feature of the work of the Liverpool team was that the entire programme was carried out without a single research grant!

As we have seen, the backgrounds and approach to the research programme of the New York team was completely different. The three scientists involved had extensive backgrounds in immunology and blood group serology and, as is clear from Gorman's account of their work,[17] they prepared themselves for the programme by a long and extensive review of the literature on antibody-induced immunodepression. The depth of their thinking along these lines is clearly evidenced by a remarkable paper, by Gorman and Chandler (published while this work was still active), on the question of whether there is an immunologically incompetent lymphocyte.[27] The team also had the advantage of Pollack's programme at Ortho, which brought very high skills in immunology and laboratory practice to the study and also had at its disposal an idle Cohn fractionation plant together with freezers full of anti-C+D antibody serum. Hence he was able to make a large quantity of anti-C+D gamma globulin for the study. There is no doubt that the New York team were a bit shaken when they heard of what was going on in Liverpool but, remarkably, there were excellent relationships between the two teams subsequently.

Did these teams have anything in common apart from a burning desire to develop an approach to controlling Rh haemolytic disease? Perhaps the only issue which they shared was the fact that experts in the blood transfusion and blood group field on both sides of the Atlantic were highly sceptical about their research and totally negative about its likely successful outcome!

10.5 Conclusions: Why Did this Work Never Receive Recognition by the Nobel Prize Committee?

Even though the precise mechanism whereby anti-D antibody protects against Rhesus disease of the newborn is still not completely understood there is no doubt that this work was one of the most important developments in preventative medicine in the second half of the 20th century. Why was it not recognised by the Nobel Committee? Presumably the answer lies, at least in part, in the number of investigators involved. As was recognised by the Lasker Award Committee, Clarke and Finn from Liverpool and the three scientists from the New York team would all have had to be named by the Nobel Committee. And careful examination of the work of the Liverpool team underlines the importance of other workers, notably Sheppard, whose critical approach to each of the developments was invaluable, as was that of Woodrow in the later stages of the programme. Also, there is Donohoe who did all the serological work in Liverpool and the invaluable help obtained from Lehane, director of the local blood transfusion service, and the obstetrician Towers, both of whom played a major role in developing the different clinical trials.

It is possible, of course, that other factors might have been involved in the Nobel Prize Committee's lack of recognition of this work. Certainly in the early days after its first successes the continued scepticism about its application on behalf of many of the experts in the blood group field was slow to evaporate. But it was clear that this approach to the prevention of Rh haemolytic disease was undoubtedly successful in the vast majority of cases long before the sad demise of some of the key investigators involved. Also, of course, it appears that different research institutions around the world vary widely in their efforts to secure international recognition and awards for their scientists. It is not clear whether this was a factor in this particular case. Overall, however, it does seem likely that the major problem was the number of investigators involved.

As is the case in much of modern medical research, increasingly large teams are usually involved and it is extremely difficult to separate the work of different individuals. Indeed, it is still not clear which member of the Liverpool team suggested the use of anti-D and we will never know.

In short, as the size of research teams increases it will be increasingly difficult for the Nobel Committee to pick out only three investigators as recipients of the Nobel Prize. This problem is particularly well exemplified in the story of Rhesus haemolytic disease and its prevention.

Acknowledgements

As in my previous accounts of the life of Cyril Clarke I am very grateful to his sons, Stephen and Charles, for details of his family. I also thank Jocelyn Morris for bringing my attention to the two monographs dealing with the New York team's work and also for putting me in contact with her brother, John Gorman, who has also helped with some valuable information and a photograph. I also thank Professor Tilli Tansey and the Wellcome Trust for their help in supplying the picture of Ronald Finn. And finally I acknowledge the invaluable help of Jeanne Packer and Liz Rose in the preparation of this manuscript.

References

1. Daniels G. *Human Blood Groups*. Oxford: Blackwell Science; 1995.
2. Zallen DT, Christie DA, Tansey EM. *The Rhesus factor and disease prevention*. Vol. 22. London: The Wellcome Trust Centre for the History of Medicine at UCL; 2004.
3. Weatherall D. Sir Cyril Astley Clark, C.B.E., 22 August 1907–21 November 2000. *Biogr Mem Fellows R Soc* 2002; 48: 71–85.
4. Weatherall DJ. Cyril Clarke and the prevention of rhesus haemolytic disease of the newborn. *British Journal of Haematology* 2012; 157: 41–46.
5. Clarke CA. Eighty-eight years of this and that: Part I. *Proceedings of the Royal College of Physicians of Edinburgh* 1995; 25: 495–508.
6. Clarke CA. Eighty-eight years of this and that: Part II. *Proceedings of the Royal College of Physicians of Edinburgh* 1995; 25: 675–687.
7. Clarke CA, Edwards JW, Haddock DR *et al.* ABO blood groups and secretor character in duodenal ulcer; population and sibship studies. *BMJ* 1956; 2 (4995): 725–731.
8. Kleihauer E, Braun H, Betke K. Demonstration von fetealem haemoglobin in den Erythrocyten eines Blutaussttriche. *Klin Wochenschr* 1957; 35: 637–638.

9. Zipursky A, Hull A, White FD, Israels LG. Foetal erythrocytes in the maternal circulation. *Lancet* 1959; 1 (7070): 451–452.

10. Finn R, Clarke CA, Donohoe WT *et al.* Experimental studies on the prevention of Rh haemolytic disease. *BMJ* 1961; 1 (5238): 1486–1490.

11. Clarke CA. The prevention of 'Rhesus' babies. *Scientific American* 1968; 219 (5): 46–52.

12. Finn R. Erythroblastosis. *Lancet* 1960; 1: 526.

13. Clarke CA, Donohoe WT, McConnell RB *et al.* Further experimental studies on the prevention of Rh haemolytic disease. *BMJ* 1963; 1 (5336): 979–984.

14. Woodrow JC, Clarke CA, Donohoe WT *et al.* Prevention of Rh-Haemolytic Disease: A Third Report. *BMJ* 1965; 1 (5430): 279–283.

15. Clarke CA, Donohoe WT, Durkin CM *et al.* Prevention of Rh-Haemolytic disease: results of the clinical trial. A combined study from centres in England and Baltimore. *BMJ* 1966; ii: 907–914.

16. Clarke CA, Donohoe WT, Finn R *et al.* Prevention of Rh-Haemolytic disease: final results of the 'high-risk' clinical trial. A combined study from centres in England and Baltimore. *BMJ* 1971; 2: 607–609.

17. Gorman JG. *The role of the laboratory in hemolytic disease of the newborn.* Philadelphia: Lea and Febiger; 1975.

18. Zimmerman DR. *Rh. The intimate history of a disease and its conquest.* New York: Macmillan Publishing Co Inc.; 1973.

19. Freda VJ, Gorman JG, Pollack W. Successful Prevention of Experimental Rh Sensitization in Man with an Anti-Rh Gamma2-Globulin Antibody Preparation: A Preliminary Report. *Transfusion* 1964; 4: 26–32.

20. Freda VJ, Robertson JG, Gorman JG. Antepartum management and prevention of Rh isoimmunization. *Ann N Y Acad Sci* 1965; 127: 909–925.

21. Schneider J. Tagungsberichte. IV. Arbeitstagung zur prophylaxe der Rhesus-sensibilisierung mit Immunoglobulin anti-D. *Geburtshilfe Frauenheilkd* 1971; 31: 493.

22. Hamilton EG. Prevention of Rh isoimmunization by injection of anti-D antibody. *Obstet Gynecol* 1967; 30: 812–815.

23. Hamilton EG. Ten-year experience with high titer anti-D plasma for the prevention of Rh isoimmunization. *Obstet Gynecol* 1972; 40: 692–696.

24. Clarke CA. *Rhesus haemolytic disease.* Selected papers and extracts. Lancaster: MTP Medical and Publishing Co Ltd., Blackburn Times Press; 1975.

25. Woodrow JC. General immunology of antibody-mediated suppression of the immune response. *Haematologica* 1970; iii: 115–117.

26. Murphy MF, Pamphilon DH. *Practical Transfusion Medicine.* 2nd Edition. Oxford: Blackwell Publishing Ltd; 2005.

27. Gorman JG, Chandler JG. Is there an immunologically incompetent lymphocyte? *Blood* 1964; 23: 117–128.

Chapter 11

HERBERT BOYER AND STANLEY COHEN: RECOMBINANT DNA

Anne Soutar

11.1 Introduction

In our so-called post-genomic era of biomedical research, it is difficult to remember that it has not always been possible to reach for a Molecular Biology catalogue and choose at will from a large selection of highly specific restriction enzymes that cut DNA at precise nucleotide sequences. Cleaving DNA with restriction enzymes produces a fragment with specific 'sticky ends' that allow its insertion into a small circular piece of DNA — a plasmid — cut with the same enzymes. The plasmid with its insert, or cloning vector as it is often now called, can then be introduced into bacterial cells where the plasmid is replicated as they grow and divide so that numerous copies of the recombinant DNA can be isolated. The original DNA can be from any species — plant or animal — and it will be reproduced faithfully in the bacterial cells to produce large amounts of the piece of DNA for further analysis. Furthermore, if the piece of DNA encodes a protein and the plasmid contains the necessary information to allow transcription of the encoded DNA to produce mRNA, the bacterial cells will synthesise the protein that the DNA encodes. This deceptively simple process has led to the explosion in our understanding of human molecular genetics and its role in human disease that has taken place in the last 20 or so years. Yet to the surprise of some, the two men behind the basic discoveries that made this possible, Herbert Boyer and Stanley Cohen (Fig. 11.1), have not been awarded the Nobel Prize for Physiology or Medicine, nor for Chemistry, despite having

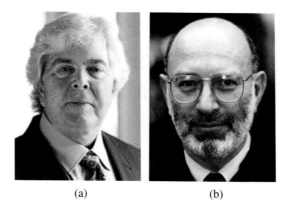

(a)   (b)

Fig. 11.1. Contemporary photograph of Herbert Boyer (left) and photograph of Stanley Cohen in 1995 (right). (By kind permission of Drs Boyer and Cohen.)

won almost every other prestigious award in the field, including the Lasker Prize in 1980 and the Shaw Prize in 2004. Both men have also been awarded the US National Medal of Science, Cohen in 1988 and Boyer in 1990.

11.2 Biography of Herbert Boyer (1936–)

From the perspective of the eastern side of the Atlantic, Herb Boyer's life story seems to personify the American Dream in that he emerged from relatively humble origins to attain both academic renown for his research and considerable wealth as the founder of Genentech, the first biotech company. Boyer has been interviewed several times to provide oral history[1,2] and in the transcripts he comes across as a charming, humorous and modest man who is pleased with but also faintly surprised by his success. In the introduction to one of these, his friend and colleague J. Michael Bishop, Professor of Microbiology and Immunology at the University of California, San Francisco (UCSF) and himself a Nobel Prize winner,[3] has described him as an incurable optimist who would embark on seemingly impossible experiments in the expectation that they would somehow work.[2]

By his own account,[4] Boyer grew up happily in a small town in Pennsylvania, son and grandson of Pennsylvania Railroad employees whose ancestors had moved to the US in 1709. Boyer says that in his early years he showed no interest in academic matters, and his life centred around football, basketball and baseball, fishing and hunting with his father — and girls. As is not uncommon, one excellent teacher, in this case his sports coach who also taught maths and science, changed his attitude and was instrumental in encouraging him to go to college. He graduated from Saint Vincent, a Benedictine college, in 1958. One career-defining event during his time was a class project that entailed him reading about Watson and Crick's newly published structure of DNA, and on the basis of the sense of excitement this generated he decided to join the graduate programme at the University of Pittsburgh to study genetics. He had failed to gain entry into medical school 'because of poor grades', but since he apparently did not realise he was supposed to pay for this himself, it was probably no bad thing. His PhD project was, in his own words, 'overly ambitious ... using microbial genetics to elucidate the genetic code. I managed to generate enough data to write a thesis on the structure of a set of related genes in lieu of my original goal, which had been solved very elegantly by others'.[4] This was enough to gain him a PhD in 1963, and, importantly, allowed him to make the interesting observation that DNA can be transferred between some but not all bacterial species. He then went to Yale to pursue this topic in Ed Adelberg's lab, where he discovered that the phenomena he had observed were based on the restriction and modification of DNA by bacteria, and he continued this line of research after moving to the University of California, Los Angeles (UCLA) in 1967 to become an Assistant Professor.

The restriction modification system (RM system), first noted in the 1950s, allows bacteria to protect themselves from invasion by foreign DNA such as bacteriophages (bacterial viruses). Certain bacterial strains were found to inhibit (restrict) the growth of such viruses grown in previous strains, an effect attributed to methylation of DNA and sequence-specific endonucleases that presumably destroyed the invading DNA without affecting that of the host. Werner Arber first suggested that restriction enzymes bound to specific sites on DNA.[5]

Boyer set out to characterise the enzymes responsible, with a particular interest in how the proteins recognised and reacted with DNA.

11.3 Biography of Stanley Cohen (1935–)

Stan Cohen's family were more recent arrivals in the US than Boyer's, settling in New Jersey in the 19th century. Cohen describes a similarly idyllic boyhood in a small American town where everyone knew everyone else, and his time was also spent playing ball games, although surprisingly he adds playing Monopoly to his list of pastimes.[6] He also developed an interest in music as he grew up, and learnt to play the piano and the ukulele. He enjoyed writing songs, one of which was apparently recorded 'by an internationally-known vocalist', but decided nonetheless that music should remain a hobby. His mother worked as an accountant/bookkeeper and his father was an electrician, so Cohen felt they were 'comfortably off' as a family. He says that, 'My father was a man of insatiable curiosity about the workings of nature, and enthusiastically supported and nurtured my own curiosity about the natural world',[6] which suggests that in his case it was his father who was instrumental in encouraging him to pursue a scientific career, although he also states that he was influenced by one inspiring teacher. Cohen was apparently torn between physics and medicine, but eventually opted to study medicine, starting with pre-medical studies at Rutgers and then moving to the University of Pennsylvania School of Medicine in 1956. Fortunately, the lure of basic science was still strong though, and he spent time after classes and during the summer recess with Charles Breedis, working on a project investigating the immunological basis of skin graft rejection. This gave him the opportunity to spend a summer in London in Peter Medawar's lab, and helped him to realise that 'investigating fundamental biological questions by laboratory experimentation'[6] was exciting and stimulating and persuaded him to pursue a career in research rather than clinical medicine. After postdoctoral positions at the National Institutes of Health (NIH) and then the Albert Einstein Institute in New York, where he worked with Jerard Hurwitz on the transcription of RNA from DNA, in 1968 he moved to Stanford

University in California as an Assistant Professor, where he remains today as Professor of Genetics and Medicine. On arriving at Stanford, as well as teaching medical students, he began his research focusing on the molecular mechanisms by which small circular pieces of DNA that are not integral to the bacterial DNA enable bacteria to become resistant to antibiotics. He 'particularly wished to know how plasmids had evolved and were propagated'[6] and his first paper on this topic was a *Nature* letter in 1969, where he described the isolation of multiple different circular DNAs from the bacterium *Escherichia coli* (*E.coli*).[7] His interest in the biology of plasmids, as these circular pieces of DNA are now known, continues to this day, as does his enthusiasm for early American folk music and playing the five-string banjo. Plasmids were and still are important for clinical medicine because they frequently carry genes that confer antibiotic resistance to the bacteria that house them and are easily transferred between different bacterial species.

11.4 Production of Recombinant DNA

Boyer was keen to find different restriction systems, and examined a collection of multiple drug-resistant *E.coli* strains isolated from patients by a colleague. Although he found that most of these shared the same specificity, one rare strain from a patient with a urinary tract infection differed from the rest. This strain expressed the RI enzyme, the other strains all expressing RII.[1] For those who routinely digest DNA with restriction enzymes and analyse the products on agarose gels stained with ethidium bromide, it is worth noting that at this time Boyer was separating digested DNA on sucrose density gradients, and that the DNA needed to be radioactively labelled with ^{32}P. He identified fragments of DNA in the gradient by collecting drops from the bottom of the tube and counting them for radioactivity. The first notable success was the identification of the recognition site for the RI enzyme he had isolated from the rare strain of *E.coli*. This was painstaking work involving the use of purified enzyme to cut a viral DNA that he had found to be cut only once by the enzyme, then filling in the cut ends with ^{32}P-labelled nucleotides and analysing the oligonucleotides produced after digesting the labelled DNA with a non-specific endonuclease to produce short fragments. He noted two key points: first, the enzyme cleaved double-stranded DNA asymmetrically to leave short single-stranded DNA ends and secondly that the recognition site was a palindrome (Fig. 11.2). He also concludes the paper reporting this finding with this statement: 'The other important feature of the RI endonuclease break is that the staggered cleavages give rise to short cohesive termini, which afford the possibility of reconstructing DNA molecules *in vitro* from any two DNA fragments generated by RI endonuclease digestion.'[8] In 1970, Hamilton Smith had published the purification and characterisation of a restriction enzyme from *Haemophilus influenza*[9] that cut DNA at the centre of a symmetrical sequence. This enzyme was used by Dan Nathans in pioneering studies to map genes in Lambda phage, work that led to the awarding of the Nobel Prize for Physiology or Medicine in 1978 to Arber, Nathans and Smith for the 'discovery of

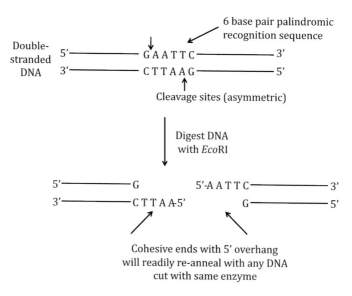

Fig. 11.2.　The nucleotide sequence of the cleavage site for *Eco*RI.

The diagram shows the 6 base pair palindromic recognition site for the enzyme and the two cleavage sites that create short ends of single-stranded DNA — 'sticky ends' — that readily allow recombination with other pieces of DNA cut with the same enzyme.[8]

restriction enzymes and their application to problems of molecular genetics'.[10] Thus a Nobel Prize had already been awarded for restriction enzymes, albeit with a very different focus to that of Boyer's work.

While Boyer was working to determine the sequence of the recognition site of his enzyme, he generously gave samples of his newly purified *Eco*RI to Paul Berg, whose postdoctoral fellows used it to cut DNA from SV40, a monkey virus containing a single circular DNA molecule that was cleaved once by the RI enzyme.[11] They found that the cleaved SV40 DNA would recircularise at low temperature, showing that the enzymic cleavage produced cohesive ends.[12] Thus Boyer was already fully aware of the possibilities for using his enzyme to produce recombinant DNA, as were Berg and others. Indeed, the gift of purified *Eco*RI from Boyer was to set Paul Berg on the way to receiving the Nobel Prize for Chemistry in 1980 for 'his fundamental studies of the biochemistry of nucleic acids, with particular regard to recombinant DNA'.[13] Boyer was trying to produce recombinant DNA during a sabbatical visit in the summer of 1972 from Bob Helling, who had been a fellow graduate student at the University of Pittsburg. However, technical problems impeded their progress until Boyer met Stanley Cohen, with whom he was to develop a fruitful collaboration.

Boyer and Cohen met at a conference in Hawaii in 1972, where they agreed to collaborate, using Boyer's enzyme to make recombinant DNA with Cohen's plasmids. During this time, Boyer describes meeting Joe Sambrook and Phil Sharp during a trip to Cold Spring Harbor to give a seminar, and they showed him how they were staining DNA fragments in gels with ethidium bromide.[1] Boyer and Helling were soon using the technique themselves and this greatly simplified their experiments. Cohen had also devised a method of treating bacterial cells with calcium chloride that made them take up plasmid DNA more readily, thus 'genetically transforming' them.[14] Their first joint experiments involved cleaving different plasmids with *Eco*RI and transforming *E.coli* with the cleaved mixture, either without further treatment or after re-ligation *in vitro*. Bacterial colonies that were able to grow in the presence of antibiotics carried a plasmid, and when they analysed the plasmids by digesting them again with *Eco*RI, they found that they had generated new fully functional plasmids.[15] They also combined two plasmids of completely different origins, each carrying genes conferring resistance to different antibiotics, to form a single new one which retained both the ability to replicate in bacterial cells and resistance to both antibiotics (Fig. 11.3). They noted that one of the plasmids, pSC101, would be particularly useful because it was small, and cleaving it with *Eco*RI left both the replication machinery and the genes conferring antibiotic resistance intact, features of cloning plasmids that are taken for granted these days.

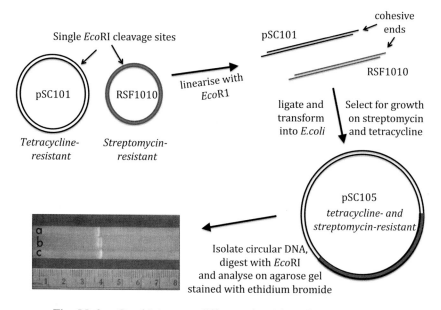

Fig. 11.3.   Combining two different plasmids to form a new one.

The diagram shows how two different plasmids, one carrying the gene for resistance to tetracycline and the other to streptomycin were cut with *Eco*RI and allowed to recombine. *E.coli* cells were transformed with the mixture and the bacteria were spread on to agar plates containing both streptomycin and tetracycline. Bacterial colonies that were able to grow carried a plasmid containing genes for resistance to both antibiotics — a recombinant DNA plasmid. When this plasmid was re-digested with *Eco*RI and the products analysed by agarose gel electrophoresis, it was found to contain fragments equal in size to the two original plasmids (lane a, original plasmid pSC101, lane b, new plasmid pSC105 and lane c, original plasmid RSF1010[15]).

The next step was to show that eukaryotic DNA — or any DNA — could be inserted into a plasmid and replicated to produce many copies. They thought it would be easy to cut up genomic DNA with *Eco*RI and insert the pieces into a plasmid, but with the techniques available then the difficulty was to select for and identify bacteria carrying plasmids with mammalian DNA inserted; the experiments recombining plasmids were relatively simple because it was possible to select for different antibiotic resistance from both plasmids. Boyer and Cohen hoped to circumvent this problem by inserting a single well-characterised piece of DNA, and for this they were fortunate to be told by John Morrow about amplified DNA encoding the frog ribosomal RNA that Don Brown had isolated.[16] Brown generously allowed them to use the frog DNA and they showed that it could be cleaved by *Eco*RI and inserted into their plasmid pSC101. They found that about 20–30% of the antibiotic-resistant colonies of bacterial cells were recombinant plasmids, each with a DNA insert that matched the size of one or more of the ribosomal DNA fragments.[17] They confirmed the identity of the inserts first by showing that the recombinant plasmids hybridised to ^{32}P-labelled ribosomal RNA, also a gift of Don Brown, and secondly by transcribing RNA from the plasmids and showing that it hybridised with ribosomal DNA, this last finding described by Boyer as 'the icing on the cake'[1] (Fig. 11.4).

Thus Boyer and Cohen, with invaluable help from others, had shown that it was possible to clone any piece of DNA such that it could be transcribed in bacterial cells. They pointed out that they did not know at this stage how accurate the transcription was or, because the DNA they had used was non-coding, whether the bacteria would make a eukaryotic protein. However, they did confirm that the cloned DNA was stably integrated into the plasmid for at least 100 generations, a fact again taken for granted today. As the authors state in the discussion, 'The ability to clone specific fragments of DNA from a complex genome provides a potentially valuable tool for the study of organization and function of eukaryotic genomes.'[17] It is likely that they underestimated quite how swiftly knowledge would advance based on this biotechnology. Everybody wanted to do it and advances in cloning techniques rapidly followed these first papers.

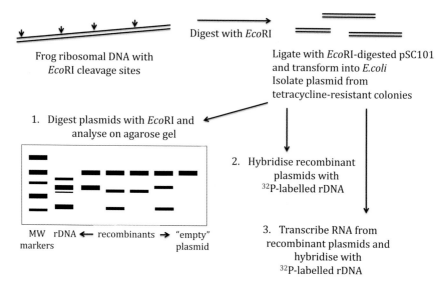

Fig. 11.4.   Cloning frog ribosomal DNA into a bacterial plasmid.

DNA encoding frog ribosomal RNA was digested with *Eco*RI and ligated into plasmid pSC101 digested with the same enzyme.[17] The ligated DNA was transformed into *E.coli* and the bacteria spread onto agar plates containing tetracycline. Colonies that grew on the plates contained plasmids with the tetracycline resistance gene, 30% of which contained DNA inserts of the expected size for frog ribosomal DNA when analysed on agarose gels (1). Confirmation that these inserts were correct was obtained by hybridising the plasmid DNA with radiolabelled frog mRNA (2) and by showing that RNA transcribed from the plasmid hybridised with radiolabelled frog DNA (3).

There was, however, one major issue that impeded progress for a while: was cloning mammalian DNA in plasmids and bacteriophages or, more crucially, in viruses, going to be safe? Leading scientists involved in the work, Boyer and Cohen included, were aware of the possible danger that if new antibiotic-resistant strains of bacteria or viruses containing 'foreign' DNA were released into the environment they could be a risk for human health or the natural environment. In 1974 they wrote a letter to *Nature* expressing their concerns, some of which had already been raised the previous year,[18] and recommended a voluntary moratorium on recombinant DNA research.[19] This was largely observed, at least in the US, but it was clear that everyone wanted to exploit the potential that recombinant DNA offered. In an attempt to resolve the problem, a conference involving international scientists, lawyers and government officials was held at Asilomar, California, in February 1975. The result of this was a set of guidelines for recombinant DNA research,[20] recommending, amongst other things, that recombinant DNA work should be carried out in appropriate containment facilities and that any plasmid or viral vectors used should be disabled so that they are unable to flourish outside laboratory conditions. Despite the many thousands of experiments on recombinant DNA that have been carried out since then, the worst fears have not been realised and, indeed, exchange of genetic material between species is now known to occur naturally.

After the moratorium was lifted, Boyer continued his research into recombinant DNA, with the aim now of producing proteins that could be used for clinical practice — for example, human somatostatin was produced in 1977 from a chemically synthesised gene.[21] One factor that may have influenced the failure of Boyer and Cohen's work to be recognised as worthy of the Nobel Prize was Boyer's co-founding in 1976 of Genentech, a commercial company set up with investment from a venture capitalist called Robert Swanson to pursue research into medical uses of recombinant DNA. This innovation was greeted with a sharp intake of breath from most of the academic scientific establishment, who felt that commercial gain was not compatible with scientific research. However, it provided support for work that might not have been supported by academic funding and Genentech went on to produce several important products, the first of which was human insulin,[22] with no apparent compromises in the quality of the research carried out. Many other small so-called biotech companies have since been set up, and many have played an invaluable role in supporting research that has brought recombinant DNA products to the point where their potential can be realised for clinical medicine. In general, promising products have been sold or licensed by biotech companies to large pharmaceutical companies that have the resources to carry out clinical trials and large-scale production, but lack the research skills to develop them in the first place. Thus the Biotech companies have remained separate from the more commercial side of the pharmaceutical industry. This is not to say that the biotech companies have not made money. Michael Bishop states[2] that Boyer 'directed all his personal income from the patents on recombinant DNA to his department at UCSF. The eventual yield was 52 million dollars, to be used for graduate education and other good purposes at UCSF — all this above and beyond the University's direct share of the patent income. A portion of the UCSF Medical Center also bears the Boyer name in recognition of an additional gift'.

11.5 How has Medicine Benefited from Recombinant DNA?

There is no doubt that the ability to clone recombinant DNA has resulted in an explosion of knowledge and understanding of human genetics and biology that has benefited all aspects of clinical medicine. Without this technique, there would be no genetic mapping, no genome sequence and no understanding of how genes are expressed and regulated. The sequence of most known proteins has been deduced from the sequence of the cDNA cloned from mRNA rather than by laborious peptide sequencing. Recombinant DNA technology has revealed the underlying cause of inherited diseases caused by single gene defects, and has allowed analysis of the structure and function of numerous proteins important in human disease. Cloned DNA can be expressed in cells that do not normally express the gene of interest, allowing the effect of a genetic variant to be determined and its role in the pathogenicity of a disease to be assessed. Detailed genetic mapping and sequencing is beginning to provide insight into the causes of complex genetic diseases such as diabetes or autoimmune diseases by identifying susceptibility genes. Pharmacogenetics, the study of the importance of individual genetic variation in the response to different drugs, is still in its infancy, but has the potential to tailor drug treatment to increase efficacy and prevent unwanted side effects. Cloning DNA is required to produce transgenic and knockout models of disease, revealing underlying mechanisms and allowing different therapies to be devised and tested. Fundamental understanding of stem cell biology and its potential for treatments involving tissue replacement has relied on expression of cloned genes. More directly, recombinant

DNA technology has been used to produce a wide variety of human proteins for therapeutic purposes, as discussed below. Gene therapy is also dependent on this technology although its full potential for 'curing' genetic disorders is yet to be realised.

The initial excitement for the medical benefits of the direct products of recombinant DNA technology was very high and expectations, it has to be said, were overhyped. In practice it took quite some time to develop products that were acceptable for use: for example, the first clinical trials of recombinant human insulin took place in 1980.[23] It should have been a safe and inexpensive replacement for the insulin isolated from pig pancreas that was then widely used, but it was difficult at first to prescribe the correct dose of the new recombinant insulin for insulin-dependent diabetics.[24] Nonetheless, today almost all prescribed insulin is of recombinant origin.

Many other products have now become available following clinical trials, such as other hormones and growth factors, including the recombinant interferons used widely as anti-cancer or anti-viral agents.[25,26] In some cases, enzymes or proteins produced *in vitro* by expression of recombinant DNA in bacteria or yeast have been used as replacements for deficiency disorders, for example, adenosine deaminase in severe combined immune-deficiency (SCID)[27] and various clotting factors for haemophilia.[28] These are of particular importance because they avoid the use of human blood-derived products with their high risk of transmitting infectious agents. In some cases, recombinant products are the only source, for example the erythropoietin (EPO) used to treat the anaemia of renal disease[29] and tissue plasminogen activator (TPA) for the treatment of stroke.[30]

Some of the most successful products have been antibodies. The genes encoding monoclonal antibodies raised in mice against, for example, a human tumour antigen, can be engineered to produce humanised antibodies that do not raise an immune response when injected into human subjects but still bind to the antigen and elicit the appropriate downstream effects.[31] Examples include TNF-specific antibodies used to treat rheumatoid arthritis, Crohn's disease and psoriasis, and EGF- and VEGF-specific antibodies for the treatment of various cancers.[32]

Early attempts at gene therapy aimed to replace the defective gene in patients with well-defined single gene disorders, for example cystic fibrosis,[33] SCID[34] and familial hypercholesterolaemia[35] by administration of the 'normal' human gene cloned into an appropriate vector. The major problem that has not yet been completely solved is efficient, safe and non-invasive delivery of the gene to the appropriate tissue or organs in such a way that its expression is sufficiently high and persistent to replace the activity of the defective gene. Many studies reporting proof-of-principle have been published, but few have resulted in effective and safe treatments, although some remain promising and many clinical trials are underway.[36] Gene therapy for severe combined immunodeficiency due to adenosine deaminase deficiency is still viable,[37] and others for which gene therapy shows promise include clotting disorders[38] and a form of congenital blindness caused by retinal degeneration for which the gene is delivered locally.[39]

Many eminent scientists believe that Boyer and Cohen's production of the first recombinant DNA is worthy of a Nobel Prize, and it would have been interesting to be a fly on the wall to observe the Nobel Committee's deliberations, as it is more than likely that their names have been discussed. Of course, prizes have already been awarded for both restriction enzymes and recombinant DNA technology, which were undoubtedly worthy, but the findings for these prizes were sufficiently different that they should not overshadow the contribution made by Boyer and Cohen. To give the last word to Michael Bishop:[2] 'As a scientist, Herb was generous with precious reagents: some say that he shipped off the makings of a Nobel Prize in mailing tubes.'

Acknowledgements

Thanks to Malcolm Parker for providing helpful comments.

References

1. Gitschier J. Wonderful Life: An Interview with Herb Boyer. *PLoS Genet* 2009; 5: e1000653.

2. Hughes SS. Recombinant DNA Research at UCSF and Commercial Application at Genentech. Available online at: *http://texts.cdlib.org/ view?docId=kt5d5nb0zs&doc.view=entire_text* (Accessed: 8 August 2013).

3. Nobel Prize Organisation. J. Michael Bishop — Autobiography. Available online at: http://www.nobelprize.org/nobel_prizes/medicine/laureates/1989/bishop-autobio.html (Accessed: 7 January 2013).

4. Boyer HW. The Shaw Prize: Autobiography of Herbert W Boyer. 2004. Available online at: http://www.shawprize.org/en/shaw.php?tmp=3&t woid=53&threeid=68&fourid=130&fiveid=117 (Accessed: 8 August 2013).

5. Arber W, Linn S. DNA modification and restriction. *Annu Rev Biochem* 1969; 38: 467–500.

6. Cohen SN. The Shaw Prize: Autobiography of Stanley N Cohen, 2004. Available online at: http://www.shawprize.org/en/shaw.php?tmp=3&t woid=53&threeid=68&fourid=130&fiveid=116 (Accessed: 8 August 2013).

7. Cohen SN, Miller CA. Multiple molecular species of circular R-factor DNA isolated from Escherichia coli. *Nature* 1969; 224: 1273–1277.

8. Hedgpeth J, Goodman HM, Boyer HW. DNA nucleotide sequence restricted by the RI endonuclease. *Proc Natl Acad Sci U S A* 1972; 69: 3448–3452.

9. Kelly TJ, Jr, Smith HO. A restriction enzyme from Hemophilus influenzae. II. *J Mol Biol* 1970; 51: 393–409.

10. Nobel Prize Organisation. The Nobel Prize in Physiology or Medicine 1978. Available online at: http://www.nobelprize.org/nobel_prizes/ medicine/laureates/1978/ (Accessed: 7 January 2013).

11. Morrow JF, Berg P. Cleavage of Simian virus 40 DNA at a unique site by a bacterial restriction enzyme. *Proc Natl Acad Sci U S A* 1972; 69: 3365–3369.

12. Mertz JE, Davis RW. Cleavage of DNA by R 1 restriction endonuclease generates cohesive ends. *Proc Natl Acad Sci U S A* 1972; 69: 3370–3374.

13. Nobel Prize Organisation. The Nobel Prize in Chemistry 1980. Available online at: http://www.nobelprize.org/nobel_prizes/chemistry/laureates/1980/ (Accessed: 7 January 2013).

14. Cohen SN, Chang AC, Hsu L. Nonchromosomal antibiotic resistance in bacteria: genetic transformation of Escherichia coli by R-factor DNA. *Proc Natl Acad Sci U S A* 1972; 69: 2110–2114.

15. Cohen SN, Chang AC, Boyer HW *et al.* Construction of biologically functional bacterial plasmids *in vitro*. *Proc Natl Acad Sci U S A* 1973; 70: 3240–3244.

16. Dawid IB, Brown DD, Reeder RH. Composition and structure of chromosomal and amplified ribosomal DNA's of Xenopus laevis. *J Mol Biol* 1970; 51: 341–360.

17. Morrow JF, Cohen SN, Chang AC *et al.* Replication and transcription of eukaryotic DNA in Escherichia coli. *Proc Natl Acad Sci U S A* 1974; 71: 1743–1747.

18. Singer M, Soll D. Guidelines for DNA hybrid molecules. *Science* 1973; 181: 1114–1119. Berg P, Baltimore D, Boyer HW *et al.* Letter: Potential biohazards of recombinant DNA molecules. *Science* 1974; 185: 303.

20. Berg P, Baltimore D, Brenner S *et al.* Summary statement of the Asilomar conference on recombinant DNA molecules. *Proc Natl Acad Sci U S A* 1975; 72: 1981–1984.

21. Itakura K, Hirose T, Crea R *et al.* Expression in Escherichia coli of a chemically synthesized gene for the hormone somatostatin. *Science* 1977; 198: 1056–1063.

22. Goeddel DV, Kleid DG, Bolivar F *et al.* Expression in Escherichia coli of chemically synthesized genes for human insulin. *Proc Natl Acad Sci U S A* 1979; 76: 106–110.

23. Johnson IS. The trials and tribulations of producing the first genetically engineered drug. *Nat Rev Drug Discov* 2003; 2: 747–751.

24. Clark AJ, Adeniyi-Jones RO, Knight G *et al.* Biosynthetic human insulin in the treatment of diabetes. A double-blind crossover trial in established diabetic patients. *Lancet* 1982; 2 (8294): 354–357.

25. Tarhini AA, Gogas H, Kirkwood JM. IFN-alpha in the treatment of melanoma. *J Immunol* 2012; 189: 3789–3793.

26. Heim MH. Interferons and hepatitis C virus. *Swiss Med Wkly* 2012; 142: w13586.

27. Hershfield MS. PEG-ADA: an alternative to haploidentical bone marrow transplantation and an adjunct to gene therapy for adenosine deaminase deficiency. *Hum Mutat* 1995; 5: 107–112.

28. Berntorp E, Shapiro AD. Modern haemophilia care. *Lancet*, 379: 1447–1456.

29. Winearls CG, Oliver DO, Pippard MJ *et al.* Effect of human erythropoietin derived from recombinant DNA on the anaemia of patients maintained by chronic haemodialysis. *Lancet* 1986; 2 (8517): 1175–1178.

30. Wardlaw JM, Murray V, Berge E *et al.* Recombinant tissue plasminogen activator for acute ischaemic stroke: an updated systematic review and meta-analysis. *Lancet* 2012; 379: 2364–2372.

31. Winter GP. Antibody engineering. *Philos Trans R Soc Lond B Biol Sci* 1989; 324: 537–546; discussion 47.

32. Leavy O. Therapeutic antibodies: past, present and future. *Nat Rev Immunol* 2010; 10: 297.

33. Prickett M, Jain M. Gene therapy in cystic fibrosis. *Transl Res* 2013; 161: 255–264.

34. Blaese RM, Culver KW, Miller AD *et al.* T lymphocyte-directed gene therapy for ADA-SCID: initial trial results after 4 years. *Science* 1995; 270: 475–480.

35. Grossman M, Raper SE, Kozarsky K *et al.* Successful *ex vivo* gene therapy directed to liver in a patient with familial hypercholesterolaemia. *Nat Genet* 1994; 6: 335–341.

36. http://www.abedia.com/wiley/index.html (Accessed: 8 August 2013).

37. Montiel-Equihua CA, Thrasher AJ, Gaspar HB. Gene therapy for severe combined immunodeficiency due to adenosine deaminase deficiency. *Curr Gene Ther* 2012; 12: 57–65.

38. Tuddenham EG, Ingerslev J, Sorensen LN *et al.* Genetic aspects and research development in haemostasis. *Haemophilia* 2008; 14: Suppl 3: 113–118.

39. Bainbridge JW, Smith AJ, Barker SS *et al.* Effect of gene therapy on visual function in Leber's congenital amaurosis. *N Engl J Med* 2008; 358: 2231–2239.

Chapter 12

HARVEY ALTER AND MICHAEL HOUGHTON: THE DISCOVERY OF HEPATITIS C AND THE INTRODUCTION OF SCREENING TO PREVENT ITS TRANSMISSION IN TRANSFUSED BLOOD

Leonard B. Seeff and Marc G. Ghany

12.1 Historical Perspectives

Viral hepatitis is a disease thought to have been known since antiquity. Reference was made to it in the Babylonian Talmud (5th century BC) and Hippocrates is believed to have referred to it as the 'fourth kind of jaundice'. In the intervening centuries to the present, the disease has been recognized largely as outbreaks during wartime, the French referring to it as '*jaundisse des camps*' and the Germans as '*Soldatengelbsucht*'. These wartime outbreaks were presumably a result of hepatitis A virus infection, spread through contaminated water and food and by close-quarter living. Percutaneously transmitted hepatitis through the use of contaminated needles was first reported in 1885 when an outbreak of jaundice was noted among German dockworkers two to eight weeks after they had been vaccinated against smallpox,[1] but whether the illness was a result of hepatitis B or C infection is of course unknown. The largest epidemic of percutaneously transmitted hepatitis occurred in 1942 when almost 50,000 American soldiers developed jaundice after having received contaminated yellow fever vaccine,[2] later clearly attributed to hepatitis B virus infection.[3] However, as the decade of the 1960s began, neither hepatitis A nor hepatitis B virus had been identified and there was absolutely no inkling that hepatitis C even existed. Indeed, at that time, viral hepatitis was considered to consist of two forms only, distinguished simply on the basis of epidemiology and incubation period — infectious (epidemic) hepatitis and homologous (serum) hepatitis.[4] Later referred to as hepatitis A and hepatitis B,[5] respectively, these diseases would become staples in the field of hepatology.

When hepatology first emerged as a distinct discipline some 60–70 years ago, practitioners could do little more than recognize the presence of liver disease (regarded mostly as a result of chronic alcoholism), describe clinical and histological features and treat a few liver disorders mainly by mechanical means, such as by withdrawing ascitic fluid or applying pressure on bleeding varices with inflatable esophageal balloons. Great strides have been made since then in identifying other liver disease aetiologies and in defining their management, predominantly by those whose focus of study is liver disease. However, some of the most important developments have come from investigators in other disciplines pursuing their own research interests, during which they have identified findings seemingly unconnected to liver disease but that have dramatically advanced knowledge of the latter. A prime example is Dr Baruch Blumberg, a geneticist, who unwittingly identified the hepatitis B virus while studying genetic polymorphisms,[6] a discovery for which he was subsequently awarded the Nobel Prize in Physiology or Medicine. In a similar manner Dr Harvey Alter, a haematologist, and Dr Michael Houghton, a microbiologist, neither of them trained hepatologists, collaborated to identify the long sought-after and equally important hepatitis C virus.

Working separately and without prior knowledge of one another, Dr Alter, a US Government researcher stationed on the East Coast of the United States, was studying post-transfusion hepatitis during which he developed carefully documented blood sample repositories drawn from both transfusion donors and their recipients, while Dr Houghton, a basic researcher in a commercial laboratory on the West Coast, was attempting to identify an agent responsible for what was then referred to as non-A, non-B (NANB) hepatitis. The two were brought together when Dr Houghton's laboratory identified what they thought was an assay for hepatitis C and immediately turned to Dr Alter for access to his uniquely well-documented blood samples. Thus the hepatitis C virus was identified, revolutionizing the specialty of hepatology and spawning a gigantic industry devoted to defining, categorizing, and eradicating this ubiquitous virus

12.2 Brief Biographies

12.2.1 *Dr Harvey Alter*

Born in New York City in 1935, Harvey Alter (Fig. 12.1) obtained his Bachelor of Arts degree in 1956 and his Medicine degree in 1960, both from the University of Rochester. His medical internship took place at Strong Memorial Hospital, Rochester, New York, and his medical residency training at both Strong Memorial Hospital and the University of Washington Hospital, Seattle. In December 1961, he moved to the National Institutes of Health (NIH), Bethesda, Maryland, where he was a Clinical Associate for four years. During that period, he conducted a research project with Dr Blumberg and was a co-author with him on the first publication referring to the Australia antigen, ultimately identified as a component of the hepatitis B virus. In 1965, he began fellowship training in Hematology at Georgetown University Hospital, Washington D.C., where he was later appointed as the Director of Hematology Research. In 1969, he returned to the

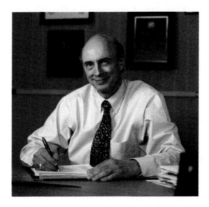

Fig. 12.1. Contemporary photograph of Harvey Alter. (Reproduced with the permission of Harvey Alter.)

NIH Clinical Center as a Senior Investigator and subsequently became Chief of the Infectious Diseases Section and, later, Associate Director for Research in the Department of Transfusion Medicine at the Clinical Center, NIH. Alter has had a close working relationship with numerous scientists conducting research on viral hepatitis at the NIH that has yielded many advances in the field. Among the many contributions to medical science made by Dr Alter, the most important include his contribution to the discovery of both the hepatitis B and hepatitis C viruses and his pivotal role in effecting the near elimination of transfusion-associated hepatitis.

Those who know Dr Alter savour his playful side and keen sense of humour. Almost every presentation he gives is accompanied by his trademark poems and/or witty slides, which have become a keenly anticipated and enjoyable feature of his talks. To this day, almost all of his communications contain some form of wordplay and this is reflected also in many of the titles of his numerous publications.

12.2.2 Dr Michael Houghton

Born in 1949 in England, Michael Houghton (Fig. 12.2) grew up in a working-class family. His father, a truck driver, became a union leader and was involved in some epic battles with Rupert Murdoch and Robert Maxwell. Houghton took the 'O' level exams at age 15 and then was admitted to a private school funded by a wealthy Shakespearean actor named Edward Alleyn. When he left for high school, his father bought him a new suit and tie with two white shirts and sent him on his way. He took the Oxford and Cambridge 'A' level examinations and won a scholarship to the University of East Anglia, which he chose because it had a good biology programme. Following that, he was admitted to King's College, in London, where he was awarded a PhD in biochemistry for work in identifying the human beta interferon gene. During this time, Dr Houghton worked with GD Searle & Co before emigrating to the United States in 1981 to take a position at the newly formed Chiron Corporation in Emeryville, California. He worked there for 25 years, during which time he focused largely on studying the virology of the hepatitis C and D

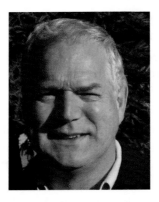

Fig. 12.2. Contemporary photograph of Michael Houghton. (Reproduced with the permission of Michael Houghton.)

viruses and trying to develop a vaccine for hepatitis C. It was at Chiron (now part of the pharmaceutical company Novartis) that his efforts led to the identification of the hepatitis C virus and the development of an assay to screen for its presence. He left Chiron in 2007 to become the Chief Scientific Officer at Epiphany Biosciences in California and in 2009 moved to Canada where he was appointed the Li Ka Shing Professor of Virology at the University of Alberta and was one of the initial recipients of a Canadian Excellence Research Chair (CERC), awarded by the Canadian government to outstanding national and international scientists. Houghton continues to work on the hepatitis C virus among other projects, including an effort to develop a hepatitis C vaccine.

12.3 The Medical Problem

Although blood transfusions to animals had been attempted in the mid-1600s, the first effort to transfuse a human was reported in 1818 by Dr James Blundell, a British obstetrician, who administered blood to a patient whom he was managing for post-partum haemorrhage.[7] Thereafter, blood transfusion as medical therapy was given only sporadically until World War II, at which time it began to be utilized on a large scale, prompting the wide-scale development of blood banks and of blood transfusion services, predominantly in the US and the UK. The occurrence of viral hepatitis following blood transfusion was first reported in 1943, involving seven patients who had developed jaundice one to four months after the transfusion,[8] and other similar reports followed.[9] Subsequently, viral hepatitis came to be recognized as one of the major and more serious complications of blood transfusion. In these early years, as already noted, viral hepatitis was thought to consist of the two forms, infectious and serum hepatitis; only later were they designated hepatitis A and hepatitis B. Because transfusion-related hepatitis was blood-borne, it was regarded as serum hepatitis and therefore believed to be caused by hepatitis B.

The ability to actually identify hepatitis B, however, took a further two decades before becoming a reality, and Dr Alter played a role in its discovery. While a Clinical Associate at the NIH Blood Bank, he was studying febrile transfusion reactions using agar gel diffusion to screen for the presence of antibodies to serum proteins in multi-transfused patients. He learned that Dr Blumberg, who was investigating protein polymorphisms at the NIH, was using the same technology. After visiting Blumberg, they began a project using agar gel diffusion and found that an unusual precipitin line developed when blood from a patient with haemophilia and blood from an Australian Aborigine were placed next to one another in wells cut into the agar gel. This line showed unexpected characteristics, one of which was that unlike lipoprotein polymorphisms where lipids stained blue, the line stained red with an azocarmine counter stain.[6] This discovery came to be referred to as the 'Australia antigen'. Additional unique characteristics were identified[10] and at first it was hypothesized to be an inherited protein increasing susceptibility to leukaemia or even a putative virus causing leukaemia. Further studies found the antigen to be present in persons multiply exposed to blood, such as those with leukaemia, and also in persons with Down's syndrome living in large institutions, and eventually its link to viral hepatitis became clear,[11] specifically to hepatitis B,[12] and a serologic assay was developed to test for its presence.

In 1967, while these events were in progress, transfusion-related studies began at the NIH with prospective evaluation of patients undergoing heart operations which revealed that viral hepatitis developed in over 30% of them, occurring, remarkably, in 51% of those exposed to blood procured from paid donors but in none of those who had received blood from volunteer donors.[13] It was at about this time that Dr Alter joined and then led the investigations devoted to transfusion-associated hepatitis, studies that have continued to the present time. A major feature of these studies is that blood samples were obtained from all consecutive volunteer blood donors to the NIH Clinical Center as well as from all their recipients. Donor blood was tested for the surrogate and/or specific virological markers existing at the time, and residual plasma was stored in −70° freezers. The recipients were screened at monthly intervals for alanine aminotransferase (ALT) levels, a marker of liver injury, as well as for the available diagnostic serologic markers, and the corresponding blood samples were also stored in the freezers. Specific criteria were established for diagnosing viral hepatitis, based largely on the development of raised ALT levels, without requiring the presence of jaundice. This was a critically important decision, because prior to that time the diagnosis of viral hepatitis was based largely on the development of jaundice and would clearly have missed many cases of hepatitis C, since most develop without jaundice.

12.4 Tackling the Problem of Transfusion-Associated Hepatitis

A series of actions were then taken with the hope of reducing the incidence of transfusion-associated hepatitis. Since paid blood donors had been identified as the primary source for transmission of viral hepatitis, the first step at the NIH Blood Bank was to move to an all-volunteer donor system. Additionally, screening of blood donors for the presence of hepatitis B surface antigen (HBsAg) began using early generation assays, and those positive for this antigen were removed from the donor list. The combined effect of these two manoeuvres was a dramatic 70% reduction in the incidence of transfusion-associated hepatitis, declining from a frequency of 33% to 9%, falling further to 6% with the introduction of a third generation HBsAg assay (Fig. 12.3).[14]

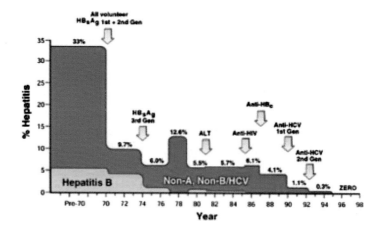

Fig. 12.3. Declining incidence of post-transfusion hepatitis in the US. (Reproduced with permission of Dr Harvey Alter.)

Retrospective screening of the stored blood samples determined that only about one quarter of hepatitis cases could be attributed to hepatitis B, the remainder being listed as non-B hepatitis. This was a surprising finding because at the time only two types of viral hepatitis were believed to exist, implying that the majority of cases of transfusion-associated non-B hepatitis cases had to be caused by hepatitis A virus infection. This unlikely consideration was however put to rest when, in 1973, investigators at the NIH identified the hepatitis A virus,[15] and testing of the non-B cases for this virus showed that none of them were positive for hepatitis A, prompting the designation non-A, non-B (NANB) hepatitis.[16] Proof that NANB hepatitis was indeed caused by a transmissible agent came soon after when Dr Alter and his colleagues inoculated chimpanzees with his NANB hepatitis blood samples and the chimpanzees were shown to develop hepatitis as defined by raised ALT values and by characteristic histopathologic findings.[17] More than a decade would pass, however, before the actual virus responsible for NANB hepatitis was identified.

When first recognized, NANB hepatitis appeared to be of limited concern because most affected persons did not develop symptoms or jaundice, and serum enzymes were only modestly elevated. However, concern began to grow when long-term follow-up studies by Dr Alter and others showed that the enzyme elevations persisted, associated with histologic evidence of increasing liver fibrosis and even asymptomatic evolution to cirrhosis.[18] Accordingly, while concerted efforts were being expended to identify the specific virus without success, energies turned to seeking surrogate measures that might be useful in identifying infectious donors and thus reduce the incidence of transfusion-associated hepatitis. Alter and his colleagues evaluated the possibility that identifying blood donors with raised ALT levels[19] or with detectable antibody to the hepatitis B core antigen (anti-HBc)[20] might be helpful in this regard. The decision to screen for anti-HBc, a component of the hepatitis B virus, was motivated by the hope that it might represent a surrogate marker for NANB hepatitis since both viruses share similar modes of transmission. These measures, however, had only a minimal impact in reducing the incidence of transfusion-associated hepatitis. Interestingly, with the introduction of these two measures, together with screening of blood donors for the human immunodeficiency virus (HIV) that began in 1985, the incidence of transfusion-associated hepatitis did decline to 4.1%. The residual NANB hepatitis cases would now have to await the finding of the responsible virus and the development of a specific test to ensure the elimination of transfusion-associated hepatitis.

12.5 The Long Quest for the Hepatitis C Virus

Cross-challenge experiments, conducted in chimpanzees, by researchers working at the Centers for Disease Control in Atlanta and at the NIH in Bethesda, using haemophilic factor concentrates and human serum known to be infectious, suggested that there might be two possible agents responsible for NANB hepatitis.[21] Taxonomic classification based on detailed physicochemical studies had narrowed the possibilities down to three virus families: *Flaviviridae*, *Togaviridae* and *Hepatitis delta virus*.[22] However, the research efforts that had been successful in enabling the discoveries of both the hepatitis A and hepatitis B viruses failed to identify the causative agent of NANB hepatitis.[23]

Enter Dr Michael Houghton in 1982, fresh from completion of his postdoctoral thesis on the cloning of the interferon beta gene.[24] Houghton had been recruited to come to the US to work at a newly formed biotechnology company, Chiron, where his task was to identify the elusive NANB hepatitis virus associated with post-transfusion hepatitis.

The effort began in earnest with a collaboration between Dr Houghton at Chiron and Dr Bradley at the Centers for Disease Control. The initial approach was a shotgun cloning strategy that involved creation of a 'cDNA library' by inserting small fragments of nucleic acids derived from infected human and chimpanzee liver and plasma (on the assumption that some clones were likely to contain nucleic acid of viral origin) into bacteria and then to screen the library using a radioactive probe that was complementary in sequence and derived from both infected and uninfected source material.[25] Between 1982 and 1986, over 25 million clones were screened, but this approach proved to be unsuccessful. Many host-derived cDNAs specific to the infected material were identified, probably representing genes involved with the host response to the chronic viral infection, but none was demonstrated to be of viral origin.[25] cDNA probes from known viruses, namely flaviviruses, togaviruses and hepadnaviruses, were used in the hope that the etiologic agent would share sequence similarity with these other viruses, but this too failed.[25] A serendipitous result of this work was the identification of the delta virus, the causative agent of delta hepatitis, another blood-borne pathogen.[26] In collaboration with Dr John Gerin of Georgetown University, the complete hepatitis D virus genome was fully characterized and shown to be closely related to plant-like viroids.[27]

Not wishing to limit himself to only a single avenue of investigation, Houghton then began to utilize a multi-pronged approach in the hope of identifying the mysterious NANB hepatitis agent. This included attempting to separate nucleic acid on electrophoretic gels loaded with chimpanzee or human liver or blood with the aim of identifying high molecular weight RNA and DNA viral genomes, culturing the organism, propagating the presumed virus in tissue culture and using electron microscopy to visualize the virus. These experiments unfortunately bore no fruit. However, as is now known, culture of the hepatitis C virus is extraordinarily difficult.

With frustration mounting and no results, a new approach was called for. The next method (and the one that ultimately proved successful) was to use a blind cDNA immunoscreening approach in which the protein product of the cloned nucleic acid is identified using an antibody rather than trying to identify the nucleic acid with a complementary nucleic acid probe.[28,29] Houghton had considered using this approach back in 1983 and 1984 but thought it was too risky because of the absence of a known specific antibody against the virus. But following a fortuitous discussion with a colleague at Chiron, Dr Kuo, who occupied the laboratory next to him, and at the suggestion of Dr Bradley at the Centers for Disease Control, Houghton became convinced that there was merit in this approach. Both of the former had recommended using sera obtained from patients with NANB hepatitis to screen a bacterial expression cDNA library in the hope of identifying a viral antigen. Critical to the success of this strategy was the availability of high titre plasma pools and liver tissue derived from the earlier chimpanzee studies conducted at the Centers for Disease Control, from which sufficient cDNA could be produced for creating the phage library. Disappointingly, the first attempt at using a phage library made from this material using chimpanzee and human sera did not yield any clones that were deemed to be of viral origin.

In 1986, Houghton received a sample of plasma from Bradley that had come from chimpanzee 910 and contained the highest titres of infectious plasma generated at that time.[30] However, using this source material for construction of the cDNA library also failed to yield any positive clones. A second phage library was then generated from plasma derived from chimpanzee 910 but this library was felt to be inadequate for screening due to technical difficulty during the cloning process. Nevertheless, after much deliberation, Houghton decided to go ahead with the screen. This time, however, he used serum from a patient with very active liver disease (believing it would contain a high level of antibody) as the presumptive source of antibody against the virus.[25] After screening over one million clones, one small clone of ~150 base pairs termed 5-1-1 was obtained which was shown to be derived from the genome of the hepatitis C virus.[31] Thus, the virus had at last been identified. To quote Houghton, 'The testing algorithm for clone 5-1-1 spanned 6 months approximately, meaning that the "eureka moment" was in fact a very gradual and extended one.'[25]

Proof that the clone 5-1-1 was derived from the hepatitis C genome was based on several lines of evidence, foremost of which was that the clone reacted with infected but not uninfected chimpanzee and human sera, and that it was not host derived.[31] This clone was used to identify the rest of the viral genome and to develop an antibody test for the virus.[32] Houghton and his collaborators christened the virus the hepatitis C virus,[31] which turned out to be a single-stranded positive-sense RNA virus with a genome of ~9500 bases.[33,34] The genome has a single open reading frame that encodes a polyprotein of ~3000 amino acids. The virus has a lipid-envelope and has been classified in the family *Flaviviridae*.[34] The entire viral genome was sequenced within one year, and antigens were expressed for the development of more specific antibody detection assays.

12.6 Final Confirmation that the Hepatitis C Virus Had Been Identified

One remaining test was needed, however, to prove beyond doubt that the antibody could accurately detect cases of NANB hepatitis. For that, Houghton turned to what were clearly the best available documented samples of NANB hepatitis, namely those that had been assembled by Alter and that included both donor and recipient material. Several sets of samples were examined under code using the developed specific assay. Among a group of 10 patients with chronic NANB hepatitis, nine were found to have received at least one donor unit positive for antibody to hepatitis C (anti-HCV) and all 10 patients seroconverted in the course of their illness.[32] Moreover, 84% of 32 patients from Italy and 78% of 23 patients from Japan with chronic NANB hepatitis tested positive for anti-HCV whereas anti-HCV was detected in only 15% of 13 Japanese patients with resolving acute NANB hepatitis. Finally, 71% of 24 US patients with transfusion-related NANB hepatitis and 58% of 59 patients with NANB hepatitis without an identifiable source were also positive for anti-HCV. The authors concluded that 'these data indicate that HCV (the hepatitis C virus) is a major cause of non-A, non-B hepatitis throughout the world'.[32] To further validate these findings, Alter and colleagues later evaluated 15 well-characterized cases from their prospective study, finding that anti-HCV developed in all 15 associated with the occurrence of the acute illness and that almost 90% of the cases had received a unit of blood positive for the antibody.[35] It is noteworthy that previous efforts to identify and distinguish the blinded and coded NANB infectious and control blood samples that had been painstakingly prepared by Alter using other potential markers had failed to break the code, underscoring the validity and importance of the current effort.

12.7 Impact of the Discovery on Medical Science

As a result of these meticulous studies, and with the introduction of mandatory screening of blood donors with assays of increased sensitivity (including nucleic acid testing at major blood banks), the incidence of transfusion-associated hepatitis in the US has fallen to a near zero frequency, as shown in Fig. 12.3. As a result, the blood supply is safer now than it ever has been.[36] It is estimated that antibody testing has prevented at least 40,000 new infections per year in the US alone and many more worldwide. In addition to linking the hepatitis C virus with transfusion hepatitis, the availability of a serodiagnostic test has enabled physician-scientists to better define the natural history of chronic hepatitis C.[37] These studies established chronic hepatitis C as one of the most common causes of chronic liver disease and cirrhosis, particularly in Western countries. The studies have also revealed a few surprising facts: ~30% of subjects exposed to the virus could clear the viral infection spontaneously without the need for treatment.[37, 38] Even more interesting, careful immunological follow-up studies of women accidentally exposed to the virus through receipt of Rhesus immunoglobulin demonstrated that many had lost their serological markers of infection.[39] Subsequent research has established a link between the hepatitis C virus and the development of hepatocellular carcinoma, essential mixed cryoglobulinemia and membranous glomerulonephritis.

The discovery of clone 5-1-1 permitted identification and sequencing of the entire genome of the hepatitis C virus. This has led to development of specific polymerase chain reaction-based assays that have been used to determine the need for and response to therapy. Understanding the life cycle of the virus and development of a cell-based replication system has led to the development of specific, direct acting antiviral agents that are potent inhibitors of viral replication, greatly improving the chances for cure of this chronic viral infection. Finally, there is a possibility that a vaccine to prevent hepatitis C may be developed in the future.

In retrospect, it is clear that the spread of the hepatitis C virus was unwittingly facilitated by advancements in medical practice, namely the development of the hypodermic needle and use of blood transfusions. Ironically, while these two advances have helped save countless lives, they have also been responsible for transmitting infectious agents to hundreds of millions of people worldwide. With regard to blood transfusions, virtually all of the transmissible infectious agents they may harbour have been identified and assays developed, so that carriers of these agents can be excluded as donors. Through the dedication and perseverance of Drs Harvey Alter and Michael Houghton, one of the most common and serious of the infectious agents, hepatitis C, has been identified and therefore no longer poses a problem for blood recipients. Moreover, their discovery extends beyond the issue of blood transfusion, having provided the opportunity to carefully study the structure of the hepatitis C virus, thus opening the way to the development of numerous direct acting antiviral drugs that have the potential of reducing or perhaps eventually eradicating this virus as a global threat.

In summary, separately and together, Drs Harvey Alter and Michael Houghton have been responsible for making blood transfusion completely safe as regards transmitting viral hepatitis, have aided in the identification of the hepatitis B and D viruses, and have been entirely responsible for the discovery of the hepatitis C virus. These accomplishments were the basis for their receipt of the prestigious Albert Lasker Award in the year 2000.

Acknowledgements

The authors wish to acknowledge the contribution of Dr Tyrrell Lorne for helpful information on Dr Michael Houghton.

References

1. Lurman A. Eine icterus epidemic. *Berl Klin Woschenschr* 1885; 22: 20–23.
2. Sawyer W, Meyer, KF, Bauer JH *et al.* Jaundice in Army Personnel in the Western Region of the United States and its Relation to Vaccination against Yellow Fever (part I) *Amer J Hyg* 1944; 39: 337–430.
3. Seeff LB, Beebe GW, Hoofnagle JH *et al.* A serologic follow-up of the 1942 epidemic of post-vaccination hepatitis in the United States Army. *N Engl J Med* 1987; 316: 965–970.
4. Neefe JR, Gellis SS, Stokes J, Jr. Homologous serum hepatitis and infectious (epidemic) hepatitis; studies in volunteers bearing on immunological and other characteristics of the etiological agents. *Am J Med* 1946; 1: 3–22.
5. McFarlan AM, Dible JH, MacCallum FO *et al.* Infective hepatitis. *Lancet* 1947; 2 (6473): 435–436.
6. Blumberg BS, Alter HJ, Visnich S. A 'New' Antigen in Leukemia Sera. *JAMA* 1965; 191: 541–546.
7. Reed EW. Selected List of References for a Study of the History of Blood Transfusion. *Bull Med Libr Assoc* 1942; 30: 242–251.
8. Beeson P. Jaundice occurring one to four weeks after transfusion of blood or plasma. Report of seven cases. *JAMA* 1943; 121: 1332–1334.
9. Morgan HV, Williamson DA. Jaundice following Administration of Human Blood Products. *Br Med J* 1943; 1 (4302): 750–753.
10. Alter HJ, Blumberg BS. Further studies on a 'new' human isoprecipitin system (Australia antigen). *Blood* 1966; 27: 297–309.

11. Blumberg BS, Gerstley BJ, Hungerford DA *et al.* A serum antigen (Australia antigen) in Down's syndrome, leukemia, and hepatitis. *Ann Intern Med* 1967; 66: 924–931.

12. Prince AM. An antigen detected in the blood during the incubation period of serum hepatitis. *Proc Natl Acad Sci USA* 1968; 60: 814–821.

13. Walsh JH, Purcell RH, Morrow AG *et al.* Posttransfusion hepatitis after open-heart operations. Incidence after the administration of blood from commercial and volunteer donor populations. *JAMA* 1970; 211: 261–265.

14. Alter HJ, Holland PV, Purcell RH *et al.* Posttransfusion hepatitis after exclusion of commercial and hepatitis-B antigen-positive donors. *Ann Intern Med* 1972; 77: 691–699.

15. Feinstone SM, Kapikian AZ, Purceli RH. Hepatitis A: detection by immune electron microscopy of a viruslike antigen associated with acute illness. *Science* 1973; 182: 1026–1028.

16. Feinstone SM, Kapikian AZ, Purcell RH *et al.* Transfusion-associated hepatitis not due to viral hepatitis type A or B. *N Engl J Med* 1975; 292: 767–770.

17. Alter HJ, Purcell RH, Holland PV, Popper H. Transmissible agent in non-A, non-B hepatitis. *Lancet* 1978; 1 (8062): 459–463.

18. Berman M, Alter HJ, Ishak KG *et al.* The chronic sequelae of non-A, non-B hepatitis. *Ann Intern Med* 1979; 91: 1–6.

19. Alter HJ, Purcell RH, Holland PV *et al.* Donor transaminase and recipient hepatitis. Impact on blood transfusion services. *JAMA* 1981; 246: 630–634.

20. Koziol DE, Holland PV, Alling DW *et al.* Antibody to hepatitis B core antigen as a paradoxical marker for non-A, non-B hepatitis agents in donated blood. *Ann Intern Med* 1986; 104: 488–495.

21. Shimizu YK, Feinstone SM, Purcell RH *et al.* Non-A, non-B hepatitis: ultrastructural evidence for two agents in experimentally infected chimpanzees. *Science* 1979; 205: 197–200.

22. Bradley DW, McCaustland KA, Cook EH *et al.* Posttransfusion non-A, non-B hepatitis in chimpanzees. Physicochemical evidence that the tubule-forming agent is a small, enveloped virus. *Gastroenterology* 1985; 88: 773–779.

23. Shih JW, Mur JI, Alter HJ. Non-A, non-B hepatitis: advances and unfulfilled expectations of the first decade. *Prog Liver Dis* 1986; 8: 433–452.

24. Houghton M, Stewart AG, Doel SM *et al.* The amino-terminal sequence of human fibroblast interferon as deduced from reverse transcripts obtained using synthetic oligonucleotide primers. *Nucleic Acids Res* 1980; 8: 1913–1931.

25. Houghton M. The long and winding road leading to the identification of the hepatitis C virus. *J Hepatol* 2009; 51: 939–948.

26. Denniston KJ, Hoyer BH, Smedile A *et al.* Cloned fragment of the hepatitis delta virus RNA genome: sequence and diagnostic application. *Science* 1986; 232: 873–875.

27. Wang KS, Choo QL, Weiner AJ *et al.* Structure, sequence and expression of the hepatitis delta (delta) viral genome. *Nature* 1986; 323: 508–514.

28. Broome S, Gilbert W. Immunological screening method to detect specific translation products. *Proc Natl Acad Sci USA* 1978; 75: 2746–2749.

29. Young RA, Davis RW. Efficient isolation of genes by using antibody probes. *Proc Natl Acad Sci USA* 1983; 80: 1194–1198.

30. Bradley DW, Krawczynski K, Beach MJ *et al.* Non-A, non-B hepatitis: toward the discovery of hepatitis C and E viruses. *Semin Liver Dis* 1991; 11: 128–146.

31. Choo QL, Kuo G, Weiner AJ *et al.* Isolation of a cDNA clone derived from a blood-borne non-A, non-B viral hepatitis genome. *Science* 1989; 244: 359–362.

32. Kuo G, Choo QL, Alter HJ *et al.* An assay for circulating antibodies to a major etiologic virus of human non-A, non-B hepatitis. *Science* 1989; 244: 362–364.

33. Choo QL, Richman KH, Han JH *et al.* Genetic organization and diversity of the hepatitis C virus. *Proc Natl Acad Sci USA* 1991; 88: 2451–2455.

34. Lindenbach BD, Rice CM. Molecular biology of flaviviruses. *Adv Virus Res* 2003; 59: 23–61.

35. Alter HJ, Purcell RH, Shih JW *et al.* Detection of antibody to hepatitis C virus in prospectively followed transfusion recipients with acute and chronic non-A, non-B hepatitis. *N Engl J Med* 1989; 321: 1494–1500.

36. Dodd RY. Current safety of the blood supply in the United States. *Int J Hematol* 2004; 80: 301–305.

37. Seeff LB. Natural history of chronic hepatitis C. *Hepatology* 2002; 36 (5: Suppl 1): S35–46.

38. Thomas DL, Astemborski J, Rai RM *et al.* The natural history of hepatitis C virus infection: host, viral, and environmental factors. *JAMA* 2000; 284: 450–456.

39. Takaki A, Wiese M, Maertens G *et al.* Cellular immune responses persist and humoral responses decrease two decades after recovery from a single-source outbreak of hepatitis C. *Nat Med* 2000; 6: 578–582.

Chapter 13

WILLEM KOLFF AND BELDING SCRIBNER: THE DEVELOPMENT OF RENAL HAEMODIALYSIS

John Turney

13.1 Introduction

If the Nobel Prize for Physiology or Medicine was awarded for innovations that radically changed the practice of medicine, then Willem Kolff and Belding Scribner would surely have been recipients, as they were of the Lasker Award in 2002. Kolff's invention[1] of a clinically usable haemodialysis machine was the first time that the function of an organ could be replaced by a machine, and ushered in the era of technological medicine which characterised the later 20th century. Scribner's seemingly simple device for facilitating vascular access[2] subsequently opened dialysis[3] to millions of patients. The contribution of both went further, changing the way that the practice of medicine was organised and understood.[4] The work of these two physicians led to a huge medico-industrial complex prolonging the useful lives of hundreds of thousands of patients worldwide, at a cost of billions of dollars each year.

13.2 Biographies

13.2.1 *Willem Kolff*

Willem Johan ('Pim') Kolff (1911–2009) was born in Leiden, the Netherlands, the eldest of five boys. He often accompanied his physician father on his rounds. An early ambition to be a zoo-keeper gave way to an interest in medicine and he graduated from Leiden University in 1937, the year that he married Janke Huidekoper (they had five children and divorced in 2002).[5] The university hospital at Groningen was the only institution willing to accept a married intern, and there he was mentored by Professors Polak Daniels and Horst Brinkman, who encouraged his early research into dialysis.

On the day of the German invasion of Holland in May 1940, Kolff was attending a family funeral in The Hague. He volunteered to set up a blood bank there, the first in continental Europe, and replicated this on his return to Groningen. Here, life under the occupation became intolerable and in 1941 Kolff obtained an appointment as physician to the municipal hospital in the small town of Kampen.[6] He negotiated technical support, which together with contacts he cultivated in the town would prove crucial in his further exploration of dialysis. His active support of the Dutch resistance to the Nazi occupation included the provision of medical certificates exempting individuals from transportation to Germany as forced labour. On occasions he administered medication to induce the appearance of jaundice, playing on the Germans' well-justified fear of hepatitis. One such recipient was Ruud Domingo, an agricultural scientist who developed a flame photometer for Kolff, later recognised as the first clinical use of rapid electrolyte estimation, essential for safe dialysis. On one occasion Kolff negotiated the release of 800 Dutch civilians being transported to Germany.

After the war, in part through Dutch émigré connections, Kolff lectured and demonstrated his machine in the US.[7] He emigrated to America in 1950, initially to the Cleveland Clinic, Ohio,[8] and then in 1967 became the Director of Biomedical Engineering at the University of Utah. He formally retired aged 75, but this in no way diminished his enquiring interest and inventiveness in devising biomechanical solutions to medical problems.

Although primarily remembered as the 'inventor' of kidney dialysis, Kolff's contribution was much greater. In the late 1950s he devised (from fly-screen mesh and a fruit juice can) the disposable twin-coil dialyser which, after refinement and marketing by Travenol of Springfield, Illinois, became the work-horse of dialysis worldwide for many years. He had noted that blood became pinker (oxygenated) during passage through the kidney machine, leading him to develop in 1955 a clinically useful membrane oxygenator ('heart-lung machine'). In 1957 he developed, and implanted in a dog, the first artificial heart. In 1982 he and Robert Jarvik designed and implanted the first human artificial heart, the recipient surviving for 112 days.

Kolff received more than 12 honorary doctorates and more than 120 international awards. Initially nominated in the 1960s, he received the Albert Lasker Award for Clinical Medical Research in 2002, jointly with Belding Scribner (Fig.13.1). He was apparently nominated for the Nobel Prize on more than one occasion. Widely regarded as the 'Father of Artificial Organs', Kolff was included by *Life* magazine as one of the 100 most important persons of the 20th century. The obituary in *The Times* stated that he 'was the supreme medical inventor of the 20th century'.[9]

13.2.2 *Belding Scribner*

Belding Hibbard Scribner ('Scrib') (1921–2003) was born in Chicago and his desire to become a physician arose during his sickly childhood. A congenital eye condition necessitated a corneal transplant in the early 1950s.[10] After graduating from the University of California in Berkeley, he proceeded MD from Stanford Medical School, Palo

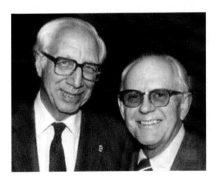

Fig. 13.1. Willem Kolff (left) and Belding Scribner (right) at the Lasker Awards in 2002. (Photograph by the late Dr Eli Friedman.)

Alto, where he was mentored by Thomas Addis,[11] one of the doyens of renal physiology. After residency at San Francisco Hospital, he became a Fellow at the Mayo Foundation in 1947. It was here in 1950 that he heard John Merrill lecturing on the use of the Kolff–Brigham dialysis machine for acute renal failure. He was appointed Director of General Medical Research at the Seattle VA Hospital in 1951 and Head of the new Division of Nephrology at the University of Washington in 1958.

Scribner was renowned as a teacher, and his clinical intelligence and thoughtful inventiveness were augmented by an ability to foster productive interdisciplinary collaboration. Over the years he influenced many young nephrologists from all over the world who went on to achieve international success. Working with visiting fellows, Scribner established home haemodialysis, developed peritoneal dialysis, and was a key influence on the science and ethics of dialysis and the clinical understanding of long-term kidney failure.[12,13]

A charismatic individual, he was known for his eccentricities: his famous red cap, living on a houseboat across the bay from the University of Washington and commuting to work by canoe. He became a connoisseur of wine and, discovering that wine was only available through state liquor stores in Washington State in the 1960s, he and friends illegally imported fine wines from California. His subsequent conviction engendered so much publicity that the state legislature passed a bill enabling the retail of wine. Bent over with osteoporosis and beset with heart problems, he drowned after falling from his houseboat. He was survived by his wife Ethel, four children and three stepsons. Scribner received honorary degrees from London and Stockholm, was President of all the American nephrological societies, and received the Lasker Award in 2002.

13.3 The Invention of Haemodialysis

13.3.1 *The science and technology of dialysis*

The artificial kidney was not invented in one place by one person but, as with all innovations, relied on an accumulation of knowledge and materials. What was required was an imaginative inventiveness to bring all the components together to create an effective therapeutic device.[4] For an innovation to be successful there has to be more than the assembling of components; one needs an understanding of the purpose and use of the device and a determination to champion its acceptance into practice. This achievement is widely credited to Kolff, but the story is more nuanced than this.

Of the many activities of the kidneys, the most obvious is the excretion of water-soluble waste products of metabolism in the urine. When this function fails, patients develop progressively worsening symptoms culminating in vomiting, coma and death. Empirically, the accumulation of metabolites correlates with the severity of the symptomatology although it is still uncertain which of the many biochemical abnormalities are actually toxic, an issue which has driven later modifications of dialysis technique and equipment, following a lead initiated by Scribner. Herman Boerhaave (1668–1738) noted the urinary odour of the internal organs of individuals dying of chronic kidney failure. In the 19th century, French physiologists identified urea and showed that it accumulated in kidney failure; it thus became known as uraemia. Urea is the most obvious, but probably the least toxic, waste product of protein metabolism and was taken as a convenient measure of renal dysfunction. Other substances have been proposed as *the* toxin but, because of the ease of laboratory measurement, urea (and creatinine) continues to be used as the indicator of the degree of renal failure and of the adequacy of treatment by dialysis. Elegant physiological studies of the kidneys continued through the early 20th century but understanding of the underlying disease processes and pathology lagged behind until immunological analysis, the electron microscope and the ability to biopsy the living kidney became possible from the 1960s onwards.

The transfer of solutes across a semipermeable membrane was discovered and named osmosis by René Dutrochet (1776–1847) in France and the science was elucidated by the Scot, Thomas Graham (1805–1869) who, when working in London, coined the term dialysis. Water and solutes move according to the concentration gradients across semipermeable membranes, the rate of transfer being determined by the size of the pores in the membrane and the size of the molecules. In dialysis machines, this transfer is influenced by other factors such as the pressure difference between the blood and the fluid of known composition (the dialysate) on either side of the membrane. The efficiency of the 'artificial kidney' is also affected by, for example, the rate of flow of both blood and dialysate or the structure of the membrane. Scribner's shunt, by opening up a mass medical market, stimulated academic and commercial research into the properties of membranes, which are now derived from industrial materials initially developed for other purposes, and into the performance of dialysis machines. Modern membranes are synthetic polymer tubes of complex microscopic structure, which are controlled by sophisticated, safe machines.

Knowledge of uraemia and of osmosis was so widely available that the early workers in dialysis barely mention it. The principle that failure of the kidneys to adequately excrete water-soluble substances led to a toxic and ultimately fatal state was simply accepted. The clinical complexities of renal failure became an issue only after Scribner's invention allowed significant prolongation of life. Thereafter, other functions of the kidneys, such as the activation of vitamin D and the synthesis of erythropoietin (essential for the formation of red blood cells), became major clinical problems which stimulated much research.

Among the many technical problems facing the pioneers of extracorporeal circuits, the most pressing was the need for an effective anticoagulant and a clinically-suitable semipermeable membrane. Contact with a foreign surface causes clotting of the blood, thereby rendering any mechanical treatment impossible. Hirudin, extracted from the heads of leeches, was an effective anticoagulant but of variable purity and with a tendency to cause febrile reactions. In 1916, Jay MacLean and William Howell at Johns Hopkins University, Baltimore, described heparin from an extract of liver.[14] Purified and standardised heparin became available in the 1930s and has remained the main anticoagulant in clinical use. A number of natural and synthetic membranes had been used experimentally in pharmacology and physiology, but all were fragile or had other problems in practice. The solution came from the packaging industry in the form of cellulose, which could be made into sheets and, eventually, tubes developed as sausage casing. Cellophane and heparin were used by William Thalhimer for experimental dialysis in 1937 in New York.[15]

13.3.2 *Early attempts at dialysis*

In 1913, John Abel, Leonard Rowntree and Bernard Turner of Johns Hopkins, performed 'vividiffusion' on dogs using hirudin and collodion tubes to extract hormones and pharmacological agents from the blood. John Jacob Abel (1857–1938) probably never intended his apparatus to be used for the treatment of uraemia.[16] Clinical haemodialysis for kidney failure was first performed in the 1920s, independently, by Heinrich Necheles (1897–1979) in Berlin (and later in Peking [Beijing]) and Georg Haas (1886–1971) in Giessen, Germany.[4,17,18] Both struggled with unsympathetic materials so that their dialysis contrivances were neither large enough nor could be used for long enough to achieve any significant clinical benefit. Nevertheless, both intended their devices for the treatment of the toxic state of uraemia.

13.4 Kolff's Invention of Effective Dialysis

In the midst of World War II, effective haemodialysis was brought to humans by three inventors, working entirely independently but with remarkable synchronicity: Willem Kolff of Kampen, the Netherlands; Nils Alwall (1906–1986) of Lund, Sweden; and Gordon Murray (1894–1976) of Toronto, Canada. Kolff is given precedence not only because he was the first to successfully dialyse humans, but also because his energetic advocacy of his new machine led to its eventual adoption, most significantly in the US, Britain and France. Alwall was a meticulous investigator, delaying the clinical use of his machine until he had completed animal experiments.[19] He faced stiff opposition in his home country, but his many publications were essential for the establishment of clinical dialysis. Murray was a brilliant, if controversial, surgeon whose contributions covered cardiovascular and other surgery, as well as dialysis.[20,21] He published little and abandoned dialysis for other projects. For obvious reasons, these three workers could not communicate until after the war: their countries were, respectively, occupied, neutral and combatant. Kolff circumvented this problem by publishing in an English-language Scandinavian journal not embargoed by the Germans. Nevertheless, not the least remarkable facet of the remarkable story of the invention of dialysis is the more or less simultaneous independent innovations, each of which provided rather different solutions to the technical and medical challenges.

Kolff later stated that his determination to invent dialysis was precipitated by the feeling of therapeutic impotence when faced with a young patient dying of uraemia at Groningen. He performed *in vitro* experiments to measure the rate of urea transfer through cellophane to enable him to calculate the length of tubing necessary to achieve a significant effect on the blood biochemistry of advanced uraemia. In this he made assumptions which were essentially proven when he tried his device on patients. Firstly, he assumed that urea, which could be both measured in the laboratory and smelled in the clinic, was a marker for whatever toxic metabolites accumulated in uraemia, causing symptoms such as coma and death. Further, if the removal of these metabolites could be adequately achieved by dialysis, this would be reflected by an improvement in the patient's symptomatology. He calculated that the surface area of the membrane and the duration of dialysis had to be much greater than any used before. He was also aware that essential electrolytes would be removed by dialysis, requiring an exchange (or 'cleansing') fluid of physiological composition. This dialysate had to be mixed by hand from available salts, which were then not necessarily of pharmacological quantity.

Present day ethical and legislative controls on clinical practice and innovation simply did not exist when Kolff and other inventors were starting the technological revolution. It has been cogently argued that dialysis would never be allowed if it had been invented nowadays.[4] Kolff's machine, assembled from available non-medical bits and pieces, did not undergo animal trials before it was used on patients and it was only at the seventeenth attempt that he was convinced that he had unequivocally demonstrated the survival of a moribund individual. Whilst the previous 16 had not been harmed by the treatment, they had not exactly been helped. This is not to say that any of the early users of dialysis behaved unethically. Without exception they were motivated, and Kolff particularly so, by a strong desire to benefit otherwise hopeless patients in any way they could. The attitudes and standards of the day allowed them to do whatever they felt to be appropriate. It does, however, raise the hypothetical question of whether modern regulatory agencies would nowadays inhibit the possible invention of radically different innovations, in the way that dialysis, mechanical ventilation or cardiac pacemakers were in their time.

13.4.1 *The first clinical dialysis*

Kolff's rotating drum dialysis machine (Fig.13.2) was an ingenious solution to a number of practical problems. By wrapping the cellophane tubing, through which the patient's blood would pass, around a large diameter drum, Kolff not only provided a large surface area for dialysis but also the rotation of the drum achieved a flow of blood without the use of pumps. The problem of the rotary coupling between the blood-lines from the patient and the moving drum was solved by using a water pump from a Ford model T engine. The

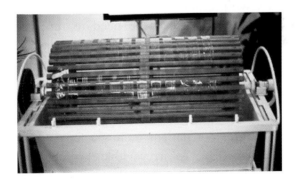

Fig. 13.2. Original Kolff rotating drum dialysis machine, c. 1945. (Author's collection.)

dialysate tank was secretly manufactured by an enamel works in Kampen. The first rotating drum was made by Kolff himself from aluminium from a shot-down Allied bomber. Thereafter, the shortage of metal meant that he had to construct later models from wood.

The first dialysis was performed on 17 March 1943, but it was not until September 1945, with the seventeenth patient, that dialysis unequivocally saved a life. Ironically, the 67-year-old patient was a collaborator who was imprisoned after recovering from her cholecystitis-related acute renal failure.

13.4.2 *The reception of dialysis*

By the end of the war, Kolff had constructed several machines which he gave to centres in Europe, Britain and America. Only at the Hammersmith Hospital, London, was a machine used, perhaps a dozen times. Despite Kolff's publications and his generosity in widely distributing both machines and blueprints, the medical profession accepted dialysis slowly. This reluctance to espouse the radical new technology had both practical and conceptual roots.[4]

The first dialysis machines were cumbersome, difficult to manage and their use was labour-intensive and fraught with danger for the patient.[21] Kolff, Alwall and others had intended dialysis to be used for chronic, irreversible, terminal uraemia (end-stage renal disease, ESRD). But one or a few dialysis treatments could at best achieve only a temporary symptomatic improvement.[22] The problem limiting the utility of the procedure was the need to repeatedly cannulate blood vessels to get a sufficient flow of blood through the machine. This vascular access was, until Scribner's invention in 1960, only possible by the surgical insertion of rigid tubes into peripheral arteries and veins. The inevitable damage to the blood vessels meant that each dialysis required a different vascular access site, limiting the total number of procedures per patient to just a few: inadequate for the lifelong treatment necessary for irreversible chronic renal failure. Thus it was only at the seventeenth attempt that Kolff treated *acute*, potentially reversible, renal failure.[23,24]

Prior to World War II, acute renal failure (ARF) had been regarded as a relatively rare, usually fatal, complication of medical crises such as complicated pregnancies. Eric Bywaters and Desmond Beall of the Hammersmith Hospital rediscovered acute kidney failure in crushed victims of the London Blitz and this triggered renewed clinicopathological analysis which came to define ARF from a myriad of causes, the cardinal feature of which is the injured kidneys' potential ability to regenerate and resume normal function after a period of inactivity. This recovery may take a few days or weeks, during which time the patient may die unless the kidney function is replaced by dialysis. Thus a 'new' condition proved suitable for a new treatment, each iteratively defining the other.

Kolff's invention directly challenged established practice and thinking. The technological revolution in medicine, which came to characterise the latter half of the 20th century, had been ushered in by a machine which, despite being difficult to use and potentially dangerous, could replace the function of a failed organ. It appealed to younger, more interventional practitioners, but was viewed with suspicion by those brought up to apply regimen: the centuries-old practice of prognosis, diet, rest and a limited pharmacopoeia. This novel approach appealed to the American post-war sense of scientific optimism, which was fuelled by the huge expansion of Federal investment in medical research and hospitals. Apart from Alwall, Europeans largely ignored dialysis, preferring instead to develop a conservative approach to the management of renal failure based on dietary manipulation of calories, electrolytes and protein. This was not entirely unsuccessful, was based on sound physiological knowledge, was not threatening to either doctor or patient, did not require special equipment or expertise, and was safe. Even in America, the acceptance of dialysis was slow and erratic. The exception was in Boston, where Kolff's machine was refined and John Merrill established the value of dialysis as part of the holistic treatment of kidney dysfunction.[25] The dialysis machine necessitated a new way of delivering medical care, the details of which were also largely worked out in Boston:[26] a specialist 'unit' staffed by dedicated physicians, nurses and technicians, at once part of but separate from the activities of a major hospital.

The dialysis machine was key to the establishment of nephrology, possibly the first of the organ-specific specialties to be defined by its technology.

It was not until the Korean War that dialysis was unequivocally shown to be effective and became more widely accepted. Deliberate US Army policy sent a Kolff–Brigham machine, manned by physicians trained in Boston, to a military hospital in Korea. The results were dramatic: the inevitable mortality in severely injured servicemen was halved.[27,28] In the mid-1950s, dialysis was started across the US, in Paris and in Leeds, UK,[29] and the number of centres performing it thereafter rose progressively (Fig. 13.3).

There remained, however, the apparently insurmountable problem of the application of dialysis to the more numerous patients with chronic, irreversible renal failure. Long-term dialysis was simply not possible without a way to repeatedly and safely access blood vessels.

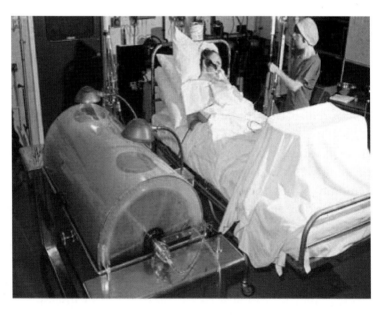

Fig. 13.3.   Brigham–Leeds modification of Kolff dialysis machine in use c. 1960. (Author's collection.)

13.5 Scribner's Shunt

As with all the early workers in the field of dialysis, Belding Scribner was frustrated by the inability to provide more than temporary palliation for patients with ESRD. The conceptually simple solution to the problem of permanent vascular access came to him following a chance encounter with a surgeon in a stairwell of Washington University Hospital. A new material, polytetrafluoroethylene (Teflon®), did not provoke a tissue reaction and so appeared to be suitable for long-term implantation. Only later did Scribner realise that it was not this characteristic but rather the slipperiness of the surface of Teflon® which prevented the clotting of blood on contact that underlay the success of his arteriovenous shunt. Teflon® was not easy to work with, but a gifted medical physics engineer, Wayne Quinton, devised a method of forming it into shapes suitable for insertion into blood vessels.[2]

Teflon® tubes were surgically inserted into an artery and vein in the wrist or ankle and stabilised by, in the early models, a subcutaneous metal plate (Fig. 13.4). The two tubes were joined so that when not in use for dialysis, the blood circulation was maintained. For dialysis, the tubes were separated and joined to the blood-lines feeding the

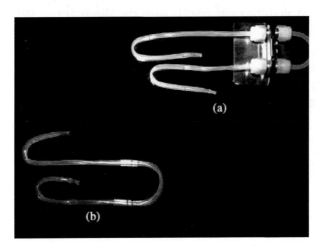

Fig. 13.4. Original Scribner arteriovenous shunts. a: Original All Teflon® cannulas with arm plate. b: All Teflon® cannulas with standard bypass. (Author's collection.)

machine. The rigidity of the Teflon® tubes proved problematic for patients in their everyday lives so, apart from the tips within the blood vessels, it was later replaced by a flexible new plastic, silastic.

Scribner's arteriovenous shunt was not a new concept: in 1948, Nils Alwall had devised and used a similar contraption for repeated dialyses. The then-available materials, such as glass and rubber, were totally unsuitable for the purpose because of their thrombogenicity. Scribner's contribution was not only to recognise the potential of newly available synthetic materials but also to harness multidisciplinary expertise, which he continued to do through a lifetime of innovation in dialysis. Despite its impact on the treatment of renal failure, the shunt was always difficult to manage. It was superseded for vascular access for long-term dialysis in 1966 by the Brescia–Cimino arteriovenous fistula.[30] By anastomosing a peripheral artery and vein, the latter enlarges and toughens so that large-bore needles can be inserted to connect the dialysis machine each time it is required, usually three times each week.

13.5.1 *The consequences of Scribner's shunt*

The shunt was a simple device with complex implications. When Scribner revealed his early results with the shunt at the 1960 meeting of the American Society of Artificial Internal Organs he was accompanied by his first patient, Clyde Shields, who lived a further 11 years on dialysis. Kolff's dialysis machine was developed to save lives; Scribner's shunt achieved the ambition of prolonging useful life indefinitely. The most immediate consequence of these developments was that the potentially huge demand for dialysis would overwhelm staff, facilities and financial resources — problems that persist today. The dilemma facing doctors, the public and politicians was that, contrary to the established model of acute care, long-term dialysis would continually add new patients to an existing cohort and so cause intensifying pressure on facilities and staff. The treatment was expensive and if it proved successful there would inevitably be exponentially increasing numbers whose medical and social needs had to be accommodated within finite resources. No precedent or robust public ethical discourse existed to guide decisions on the allocation or rationing of this life-saving treatment.[31] Scribner's response was to arrange for an independent committee of lay persons to assess the 'suitability' of potential applicants for the scarce places on the Seattle dialysis programme. This overt rationing of care on social as well as medical grounds caused a furore, but has been widely regarded to have been the start of the concept and practice of the discipline of medical ethics.[32]

Long-term dialysis revealed a host of difficulties, both technical and clinical. Scribner worked with associates and with industry to produce safer, more efficient machines that would be manageable by patients themselves at home or in renal units, which could be staffed by nurses and technicians. He identified and sought to ameliorate the medical complications which plagued the lives of ESRD patients kept alive for years by regular dialysis: disorders of the nervous and cardio-vascular systems, of bones and also chronic anaemia.[33] The Seattle group were the first to identify these problems and made important contributions to their technical and therapeutic solutions. Scribner remained a forceful advocate for his patients, and was an important mover in the 1972 amendment to Medicare which made dialysis universally available in the US, irrespective of the ability to pay.

13.6 The Impact of Kolff and Scribner on Medical Science

Most Nobel Prizes for Physiology or Medicine have been awarded to laboratory scientists, for whose work there has been but limited translation from bench to bedside. In this regard, the Nobel Prizes have reflected the emphasis on funding of 'basic' science by universities and governments. Willem Kolff and Belding Scribner were entirely different. Although both had impeccable academic credentials, they preferred to subsume their scientific knowledge in the pursuit of practical technical solutions to pressing clinical needs. In other words, their inestimable contributions were to clinical medicine and not to physiology, although their innovations opened up a huge field of scientific enquiry. Without exaggeration they were pioneers: they entered uncharted territory and by so doing, and with a singleness of purpose, they changed the face of medical practice.

There was no way that Kolff could have foreseen the consequences of his initial attempt at clinical dialysis. It was the first instance of the modern era of technological medicine. To be successfully applied, the machine necessitated a rethink of the pathogenesis and clinical consequences of diseases of an entire organ system. To be properly exploited, the machine required a new breed of specialist physicians, nurses, technicians and support staff. For efficient management, the machine and its attendants had to be housed in newly created 'units', thereby gaining status in the medical hierarchy and setting a pattern for a process repeated as other specialties arose in the second half of the 20th century. Fundamentally, Kolff offered a new way of thinking: that the function of a failed organ could be replaced mechanically, thereby postponing or preventing inevitable premature death. Although a number of individuals worked alone on the same grand project, Kolff stands out from the rest because of his persistent inventive genius and his determination, which brought his devices to the medical world where they could be developed and refined for the benefit of many. Kolff built on the work of others and did not introduce or refine some of the essential elements of the machine. He is regarded as the central figure in the development of dialysis because he made the technical, conceptual and social connections that established its usefulness. That modern sophisticated computerised dialysis machines bear little external resemblance to Kolff's leviathan is irrelevant: they perform the same function using the same principles that he demonstrated in war-torn Holland.

Scribner's shunt had even more far-reaching consequences. The ingenious little device gave hope of prolonged useful life to countless individuals worldwide. At last the promise of Kolff's machine could be realised. Scribner's character and intellect enabled him to identify and then address the implications of his actions by continued ethical, political and clinical scientific endeavour. Scribner understood that his little gadget had opened a new era in which technological medicine had properly arrived and could be applied to the masses over long periods. With it had come new clinical, fiscal, political and behavioural challenges, to the solution of which he contributed immensely. If citations are a measure of impact, then Scribner was the most influential nephrologist of his, and possibly any, generation.

The counterfactual proposal that the many achievements of Kolff and Scribner should have been recognised by the Nobel Committee is indicative of the injurious divide pervading modern medicine and clearly apparent in nephrology: the division between science and clinical practice. Innumerable patients and their families, as well as all those involved in the delivery of renal care, would heartily endorse their nomination as recognition of their immeasurable contribution to medicine. However, whatever their pragmatic successes, this was not science as presently recognised but instead was regarded by many as merely empirical problem-solving. As Kolff himself modestly observed, 'there was nothing about the machine that someone with an elementary knowledge of science could not understand'.[4] It was many years before national and international renal societies would accept studies related to dialysis on the grounds that it was treatment and had little scientific merit. This forced those involved in the practical arm of the specialty to form their own separate professional societies and registries. Despite the wealth of clinical research that eventually went into the theory and mechanics of dialysis and into the disease burden suffered by its patients, there remained a feeling in some academic quarters that this remained 'not science'. It is telling that when Kolff and Scribner achieved recognition in old age by receiving the Lasker Award, it was for *clinical* medical research, and not for basic medical science. The much misquoted phrase of Bernard of Chartres (died c. 1130), paraphrased by Isaac Newton, applies particularly to Kolff and Scribner: it was on the shoulders of these giants that modern technological medicine, with all its challenges and complexities, was built.

References

1. Kolff, WJ, Berk HTJ, ter Welle M *et al.* The artificial kidney: a dialyser with great area. *Acta Med Scand* 1944; 117: 121–134.

2. Quinton W, Dillard D, Scribner BH. Cannulation of blood vessels for prolonged hemodialysis. *Trans ASAIO* 1960; 6: 104–113.

3. Scribner BH, Buri R, Caner JEZ *et al.* The treatment of chronic uremia by means of intermittent hemodialysis: a preliminary report. *Trans ASAIO* 1960; 6: 114–122.

4. Cameron JS. *A History of the Treatment of Renal Failure by Dialysis.* Oxford: Oxford University Press; 2002.

5. Heiney P. *The Nuts and Bolts of Life: Willem Kolff and the Invention of the Kidney Machine.* Stroud: Sutton; 2002.

6. van Noordwijk J. *Dialysing for Life: The Development of the Artificial Kidney.* Dordrecht: Kluwer; 2001.

7. Kolff WJ. First clinical experience with the artificial kidney. *Ann Intern Med* 1965; 62: 608–619.

8. Kolff WJ. The early years of artificial organs at the Cleveland Clinic: Part 1: Artificial kidney and kidney transplantation. *ASAIO J* 1998; 44: 3–11.

9. Anon. Obituary. *The Times* 2009; 18 February: 34.

10. Blagg CR. Belding Scribner interviewed. *Nephrology* 1998; 4: 295–297.

11. Peitzman SJ. Thomas Addis (1881–1949): mixing patients, rats, and politics. *Kidney Internat* 1990; 37: 833–840.

12. Blagg CR. The early years of chronic dialysis: the Seattle contribution. *Nephrology* 1998; 4: 235–238.

13. Blagg CR. The early history of dialysis for chronic renal failure in the United States: a view from Seattle. *Amer J Kid Dis* 2007; 49: 482–496.

14. Marcum JA. The development of heparin in Toronto. *J Hist Med Allied Sci* 1997; 52: 310–337.

15. Cameron JS. Practical haemodialysis began with cellophane and heparin: the crucial role of William Thalhimer (1884–1961). *Nephrol Dial Transplant* 2000; 15: 1086–1091.

16. George CRP. John Jacob Abel reinterpreted: prophet or fraud? *Nephrology* 1998; 4: 217–222.

17. Wizemann V, Ritz E. Georg Haas: A forgotten pioneer of haemodialysis. *Nephrology* 1998; 4: 229–234.

18. George CRP. Hirudin, heparin and Heinrich Necheles. *Nephrology* 1998; 4: 225–228.

19. Alwall N. Historical perspective on the development of the artificial kidney. *Artif Organs* 1986; 10: 86–99.

20. Heimbecker RO. The Gordon Murray story. *Trans ASAIO* 1983; 29: 454–455.

21. Peitzman SJ. Science, inventors and the introduction of the artificial kidney in the United States. *Sem Dialysis* 1996; 9: 276–281.

21. Kolff WJ. The beginning of the artificial kidney. *Artif Organs* 1993; 17: 293–299.

23. Kolff WJ. The artificial kidney — past, present, and future. *Circulation* 1957; 15: 285–294.

24. Peitzman SJ. *Dropsy, Dialysis and Transplant.* Baltimore: Johns Hopkins University Press; 2007.

25. Swann RC, Merrill JP. The clinical course of acute renal failure. *Medicine (Balt)* 1953; 32: 215–292.

26. Merrill JP. Early days of the artificial kidney and transplantation. *Transplant Proc* 1981; 13: Suppl 1: 4–8.

27. Smith LH, Post RS, Teschan PE *et al.* Post-traumatic renal insufficiency in military casualties. II. Management, use of an artificial kidney, prognosis. *Amer J Med* 1955; 18: 189–198.

28. Teschan PE. Acute renal failure during the Korean war. *Renal Failure* 1992; 14: 237– 239.

29. Turney JH, Blagg CR, Pickstone JV. Early dialysis in Britain: Leeds and beyond. *Amer J Kid Dis* 2011; 57: 508–515.

30. Konner K. History of vascular access for haemodialysis. *Nephrol Dial Transplant* 2005; 20: 2629–2635.

31. Scribner BH. Ethical problems of using artificial organs to sustain human life. *Trans ASAIO* 1964; 10: 209–212.

32. Scribner BH. A personalized history of chronic hemodialysis. *Amer J Kid Dis* 1990; 16: 511–519.

33. Jonsen AR. *The Birth of Bioethics.* New York: Oxford University Press; 1998.

Chapter 14

JAMES TILL AND ERNEST McCULLOCH: THE DISCOVERY OF STEM CELLS

Joe Sornberger

14.1 Introduction

Discovery is a difficult word. Did Italian Christopher Columbus discover America near the end of the 15th century on his failed attempt to find a quicker route to the East Indies for his Spanish patrons? Leif Eriksson, who came ashore in Newfoundland half a millennium earlier, might have something to say about that. And what of the hundreds of thousands of indigenous people that Columbus misnamed Indians who had inhabited their lands for thousands of years?[1]

Did James Edgar Till and Ernest Armstrong McCulloch discover stem cells? Long before this improbable pair began working together in the newly created Ontario Cancer Institute in Toronto in the late-1950s, many had theorized that some kind of master, precursor cell existed. What Till and McCulloch did was prove the existence of the stem cell in a series of exquisitely executed experiments that — to this day — define its properties: (1) the ability to differentiate into clonal colonies of specialized cells and (2) the capacity to self-renew to perpetuate the differentiation process. Transplanting bone marrow in mice, they took what others had pondered and produced the functional assays that provided quantitative proof of what a stem cell does. So while they never presented the world with a glass microscope slide of a single stem cell — which might be why they never won the Nobel Prize — they did what the Lasker Foundation called 'ingenious experiments that first identified a stem cell — the blood-forming stem cell — which set the stage for all current research on adult and embryonic stem cells'.[2] If that isn't discovery, what is?

14.2 Biographies

They say that opposites attract. Till and McCulloch are proof of that. They came from entirely different social backgrounds, different geographies, and appreciated very different things.

14.2.1 *James Till*

Though now in his 80s, Till can often be found in his office at Toronto's Princess Margaret Hospital, taking public transit to get there and back. He is a tall man who is still as rakishly handsome as he is rigorously humble. Circumspect, he eschews exaggeration and offers opinions only on topics he has considered carefully. He can, however, get animated about curling, the only sport that captured his imagination as wholly as did the field of biophysics. (He twice took part in experiments to assess the impact of sweeping on the trajectory of a curling stone.) The son of a homesteader, Till was raised on an Alberta farm on the Canadian Prairies where, as a youth, he did mental time-in-motion studies while bundling sheaves of wheat into stooks for the thresher, displaying not only a keen mind but an extraordinary capacity for hard work:

> We worked from five in the morning until nine in the night. We had one quarter section that was all one field, all planted to wheat. It was cut and my job was to stook it. I remember looking at one hundred and sixty acres of sheaves and thinking, 'I've got to stand all those on end!' But you just do it. You just lean in and do it.[3]

Scholarship money secured him a place at the University of Saskatchewan in Saskatoon where, as a graduate student in the early 1950s, he came under the influence of Harold Elford Johns. A pioneer of the Cobalt bomb radiation treatment for cancer, Johns was once described as 'almost ruthless with those who did not measure up, especially those who did not demonstrate a proper work ethic'.[4] Johns encouraged Till to try his hand at biophysics, which became the focus of his PhD studies at Yale (once again thanks to scholarship money — this time provided by the National Cancer Institute of Canada). Upon receiving his doctorate in 1957, Till declined the post of Assistant Professor with the Ivy League institution and opted to do his postdoctoral work in Toronto (Fig. 14.1) with Lou Siminovitch, a microbiologist who had returned to Canada from the Louis Pasteur Institute in France, for one year while the Ontario Cancer Institute (OCI) was being built.

14.2.2 *Ernest McCulloch*

McCulloch was born into prosperity in Toronto in 1926. The son of a doctor, he was nicknamed 'Bun' while still in the cradle — a label,

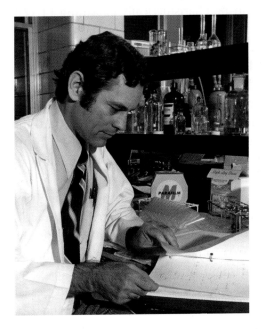

Fig. 14.1. James Edgar Till, a former prairie farm boy who turned down a teaching post with Yale to work at the Ontario Cancer Institute in Toronto, brought his biophysics expertise and rigorous attention to detail to the partnership with McCulloch. (Courtesy of the University Health Network.)

try as he might, he could never successfully shake off. Not dependent on scholarship funds for his schooling, he attended Upper Canada College where Toronto's upper crust sends its scions to become the next masters of business and the professions. No wheat-stooking for him, McCulloch spent his summers at the family's place in the country, where he learned to sail.

While McCulloch, who died in early 2011, enjoyed a privileged life, he was anything but elitist. He described the Toronto of his youth as a mean-spirited and anti-Semitic place that only became more tolerant and tolerable after the influx of immigration in the second half of the 20th century.[3] His love of literature led him to memorize long passages of poetry — he wooed his wife by quoting Alfred Lord Tennyson's 'Ulysses'[5] — and was as familiar with the works of William Shakespeare and Anthony Trollope as he was with James Blundell and Louis Pasteur. The short, stout and balding McCulloch could be charismatically charming (T-cell discoverer Tak Wah Mak said he would walk into the path of an oncoming bus for his mentor McCulloch) as he could be coldly cruel (he once advised a visiting postdoctoral fellow who had just finished a presentation to burn all his slides).[3]

McCulloch followed in his father's footsteps by taking up medicine, earning his MD at the University of Toronto in 1948 and, with it, an opportunity for a year's study at the Lister Institute in London, England — an experience that awakened in him a yearning to do medical research. Returning to Canada, he worked at Toronto General Hospital and Sunnybrook Hospital through 1953, specializing in internal medicine and establishing a medical practice. All the while, though, he was also doing research with the Banting Institute and becoming an expert in haematology. After he joined the University of Toronto's Department of Medicine in 1954, his patient roster began to dwindle as he spent more time in laboratories and lecture halls (Fig. 14.2). 'A medical practice is a business and I have never had a head for business,' he declared.[3] His acceptance of the post of Head of Haematology in the Biology Division at the brand new OCI in 1957 signalled the end of his private practice and positioned him for what would become his remarkable research partnership with Till.

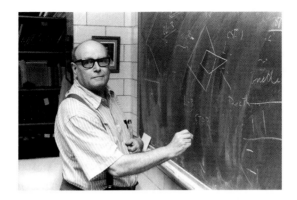

Fig. 14.2. Ernest Armstrong 'Bun' McCulloch was a clinician turned researcher who noticed the bumps on the spleens of mice and correlated them to the number of transplanted bone marrow cells (about 10,000 to 1) leading to elegant and enduring assays that proved the existence of stem cells. (Courtesy of the University Health Network.)

14.3 Setting the Stage for Stem Cell Discovery

Radiation therapy had come a long way since its beginnings around the turn of the 20th century. For decades, physicians used X-rays or implanted radium near tumours to kill cancer cells, but the treatments were complicated, costly and not especially effective. The introduction of reliable radiation delivery systems in the early 1950s, particularly Johns' Cobalt bomb, and the availability of the more potent and affordable Cobalt-60 isotope, produced in volume at Ontario's Chalk River nuclear facility, meant oncologists could attack cancer more vigorously, including previously deep-set tumours in the bladder, cervix and lungs.[6]

In the late-1940s, American Leon O. Jacobson had been irradiating mice whose protruding spleens were encased in lead, demonstrating that they could survive and rebuild their blood supply while ordinary irradiated mice could not. Jacobson theorized that the spleen contained some kind of recovery factor. It should be noted that this work was driven not by the desire to cure cancer but by the potential doomsday scenario posed by the threat of nuclear war. In her 2009 paper,

Manhattan Transfer: Lethal Radiation, Bone Marrow Transplantation, and the Birth of Stem Cell Biology, c. 1942–1961, Alison Kraft documents how Jacobson and his colleague Egon Lorenz originally studied the effects of radiation on the blood system in an attempt to find treatments for 'radiation sickness' in the event of a nuclear attack, but that 'in the course of this research it became apparent that within the bone marrow there was an "active principle," the means to regenerate the blood system'.[7] Jacobson got it wrong, however, believing the recovery trigger was hormonal rather than cell-based, as a prominent group of British biophysicists, led by Charles Ford, John Freeman Loutit and D.W.H. Barnes, proved in the 1950s.[8] Bone marrow transplantation as a treatment for leukaemia emerged from this line of thought. The earliest efforts, however, including one in Regina, Saskatchewan, and six by eventual Nobel laureate E. Donnall Thomas, which he reported on in 1957, were failures.

14.4 The Discovery of Stem Cells

It was against this background that Till and McCulloch began their work. Till can't remember when he met McCulloch, but recalls listening to him give a talk about his plans to irradiate mice and thinking it was interesting. McCulloch said it was Johns, Till's old Master's advisor who had become head of the OCI's Physics Division, who teamed them up:

> Harold's reputation was built on accurate measurements of radiation; he wasn't going to have any damn biologist ruining his reputation by misusing his machines. Jim volunteered to be the radiation expert and keep me on the straight and narrow. As soon as we got together, we found we worked well together.[3]

14.4.1 The 'Eureka!' moment

Till and McCulloch focused their work on the sensitivity of bone marrow cells to ionizing radiation for potential applications in cancer treatment. 'Because the limiting factor in cancer treatment is the sensitivity of normal tissue,' explains Till, 'you want a differential effect on the tumour.'[9] In the course of carrying out this work, McCulloch returned to the laboratory on Sunday afternoon in 1960 to check for variations in growth patterns among mice that, 10 days earlier, had been exposed to full-body radiation and injected with either irradiated or normal bone marrow cells. Some time later McCulloch would realize no such variations occurred,[10] but on that day something else intrigued him: there were bumps on the spleens. Looking closer, he realized there was a direct correlation: the more marrow cells transplanted, the more bumps on the spleens — a ratio that worked out to be about 10,000 cells per bump. Till remembers the 'Eureka' moment:

> I recall him coming along waving a piece of graph paper on which he had plotted the number of bumps versus the number of marrow cells transplanted. He said, 'You've got to see this!' We were so intrigued by this that we abandoned all the experimental research we had been doing ... and concentrated on finding out about the bumps. After about two years of hard work we were able to show that the bumps were formed by individual transplanted cells that had landed at random in the spleen and ... had proliferated and given rise to blood-forming cells. It actually solved the problem that had been around in experimental haematology since the early 1900s, which was: are the different specialized cells of the blood — red cells, white cells — descended from separate stem cells, each having its own, or can more than one kind of specialized cell come from the same stem cell? The evidence that we were able to obtain, from looking at these lumps, showed that it was the latter.[11]

14.4.2 *Colony-forming units*

Till's comment that the Sunday afternoon discovery led to 'two years of hard work' illustrates both his cautious nature and the partners' rigorous attention to detail. In the paper that emerged from the 1960 observations of the bumps on the spleens, published in February of 1961 in the niche — some would say obscure — journal called *Radiation Research*, Till and McCulloch did not use the term 'stem cells'. Instead, they called the marrow cells that were capable of making specialized blood cells 'colony-forming units' or CFU-S.

They did this, as McCulloch wrote in his book about the OCI, after much discussion 'on the nature of the entity that gave rise to each colony' and even though their calculations showed 'what would be expected if only one thing gave rise to each nodule [bump] in the spleen'.[10]

Their 1961 paper, A Direct Measurement of the Radiation Sensitivity of Normal Mouse Bone Marrow Cells, has been cited more than 3,600 times[12] and is widely regarded as the starting point for stem cell science. Stanford University's Irving Weissman, who would go on to be the first to purify both murine and human blood stem cells, described how finding out about the paper was one of those thunderbolt moments in a person's life that 'is so important you remember it in startling detail'. He wondered, 'if I would have been astute enough to follow it up rather than trashing the finding as some artifact or infection'.[13]

More than 50 years later, however, the ever-understated and understating Till is almost dismissive of the first effort, saying, 'by itself, I don't think it proved anything. We just said the cells that could form colonies in the spleen had the properties you would expect of stem cells'.[9]

14.4.3 *Search for the single cell*

McCulloch, too, thought the 1961 paper merely got things started and that 'the value of the spleen colony method depended on determining if a CFU was a single cell or several cells acting together'.[10] In addressing that challenge, they were helped out by colleagues in the UK who had proved it was possible to produce chromosomal markers among the repopulating cells in bone marrow. Charles Ford from Harwell gave a seminar at the OCI at which Till and McCulloch realized that the technique could be applied to trace the CFU-S back to their roots. Andrew Becker, a medical doctor and doctoral student working with Till, undertook this work. The process turned out to be particularly painstaking, requiring several months of arduous effort. For his work Becker earned lead author status on the 1963 *Nature* paper that demonstrated that the colonies found in the spleen of various clone cells that originated in a single cell populated the lumps:

> Since normal mouse marrow contains no uniquely and uniformly marked colony-forming cell aggregates, and since chromosome breakage by radiation is a random process, rendering highly improbable the generation of an identical abnormality in each of the cells of a hypothetical colony-forming aggregate, it can be concluded that all the cells in these marked colonies were derived from a single cell in which a chromosome aberration was induced by radiation.[14]

14.4.4 *The missing piece — self-renewal*

As with the 1961 paper, the words 'stem cell' do not appear in the *Nature* report. Despite demonstrating clonality and single-cell generation of multiple specialized cells, they felt they hadn't gone far enough in making the case for stem cells. The missing piece was proof that the precursor cells had the power to renew themselves. They found it when they collaborated with Lou Siminovitch, the geneticist who had been Till's postdoctoral advisor when he returned to Canada from Yale. Siminovitch led the experiment, designed to test what happened when the bumps were separated into their various cellular parts and re-transplanted into other irradiated mice. The paper, also published in 1963 but this time in the *Journal of Cellular Physiology*, established that the CFU-S could self-renew. Thus assured, they finally employed the term 'stem cell' — although not in the paper's title.[15]

'That's where we first used the term and where we provided the definition,' says Till. 'At that time, there was no functional definition for stem cells. We wrote it and it's still being used. That's the most lasting achievement, probably.'[9]

One other paper might also be noted: a Till-led exercise that used stochastics, which, in essence, integrates a degree of randomness into statistical calculations, to account for the distribution of the CFU-S in spleen colonies. A degree of randomness, Till argued, ought to be expected when cells are choosing whether to renew or differentiate.[16] His work, however, was criticized, particularly by John J. Trentin from the Division of Experimental Biology at Baylor College of Medicine in Houston, Texas, who contended that bone marrow stems cells' fate is the product of 'hemapoietic inductive microenvironments'.[17] Till shrugged it off:

> I found it kind of amusing. Biologists have a problem with randomness. They think deterministically. They don't like probability. Whereas someone with a physics background, especially if they've studied quantum theory or even nuclear decay, is accustomed to randomness that's mind-boggling.[3]

14.5 The Role of Stem Cells in Bone Marrow Transplantation

Bone marrow transplantation, which took more than a decade to become clinical practice after failed attempts in the mid- to late-1950s, is the most obvious — and successful — application of stem cell science. However, as previously noted, Thomas and others were already at work on transplanting bone marrow before Till and McCulloch provided their assays that proved the existence of stem cells and defined their properties.

Rainer Storb, who joined the Thomas team in the mid-1960s, says the early efforts were inspired by evidence that 'showed that when you rescued lethally irradiated mice with a spleen cell or a marrow transplant, the rescue was accomplished by cellular elements, by a cell or cells that contributed to the repopulation of marrow spaces'. He refers to work published by Joan M. Main and Richmond T. Prehn of the US National Cancer Institute, Loutit and Barnes with the Harwell group, and Holland's Dirk van Bekkum as 'what triggered the clinical effort'.[3]

However, the impact of the discovery on bone marrow transplantation should in no way be underestimated. 'It was the intellectual underpinning for our work,' says Storb. 'The concept of transplantable marrow cells that were self-replicating was already there at that time. Till and McCulloch's contribution was to document that this originated truly in a single cell. It was a very helpful piece of work. It showed that it's a hierarchal system.'[3]

When Till and McCulloch were awarded the Albert Lasker Award for Basic Medical Research in 2005, Evelyn Strauss made the contribution apparent:

> By the early 1970s, Till and McCulloch's experimental observations were clear-cut: They revealed that bone marrow transplantation owes its restorative powers to a single type of cell that not only can divide, but can differentiate into all three types of mature blood cells — red cells, white cells, and platelets. These features meant that the colony-forming cells represented a new class of progenitor cells — ones that could proliferate enough to repopulate the bone marrow of an entire animal, self-renew, and give rise to specialized cells that have limited life spans. This definition of a stem cell still holds true today.[2]

14.6 Precursor versus Stem Cell

Till and McCulloch indeed did write the definition of stem cells in their Siminovitch-led 1963 paper and it has stood the test of time. In fact, the notion of what a stem cell is has been so incorporated into the medical body of knowledge, it is simply taken for granted. What is forgotten is that two Canadians, hard at work in Toronto's Ontario Cancer Institute, proved it more than 50 years ago.

There is also the argument that what Till and McCulloch were working with were not true stem cells but precursor cells whose stem cell origins went further back. And there is merit in that debate. Norman Iscove, who worked closely with McCulloch when 'Bun' began the Princess Margaret Hospital's bone marrow transplantation program in the early 1970s, has published on the subject and, in an obituary for McCulloch published in *Cell Stem Cell* in 2011, clarified things:

> Although McCulloch and Till came to consider CFU-S to be 'stem cells' they did not explicitly equate the CFU-S with durable reconstituting stem cells and considered the possibility that CFU-S and lymphoid precursors might share a more primitive ancestor. [Wu *et al.*[18]] Later work did indeed establish the distinction between CFU-S and more primitive cells capable of systemic reconstitution ... affirming the wisdom of their inclination to use operational rather than conceptual nomenclature in describing experimental work with incompletely characterized precursor cells.[19]

Context here is crucial. Till and McCulloch were doing their work in the pre-computer, pre-digital, pre-information technology era. They were plotting their results in pencil on graph paper. More importantly, they were toiling in the dark. As Weissman has pointed out, much of what we now assume in the field of haematology was unknown then. What Till and McCulloch did, he says, 'was to turn thinking around from, "The bone marrow is a black box; we don't know anything about it", to, "The bone marrow has discrete cells that can make multiple different cell types."'[3]

Indeed the true refinement of the 'pure' human haematopoietic stem cell would take 50 years to accomplish and, fittingly, it was John E. Dick, a Till and McCulloch research descendant at the OCI, whose lab achieved it.[20]

14.7 The Discovery of Embryonic Stem Cells

Till and McCulloch worked exclusively in the field of adult stem cells and, within those parameters, were focused on blood-based stem cells. In fact, the isolation of the human embryonic stem cell by James Thomson of the University of Wisconsin in 1998 had little to do with them. The origins of that work, according to Gail Martin, the American researcher who coined the term 'embryonic stem cell', can be traced to investigations into the properties of teratoma tumours begun by Leroy Stevens in the 1950s at the Jackson Laboratory in Maine.

> What he discovered was that these tumours came from primordial germ cells that began to proliferate in an abnormal way in the embryonic testis and then developed into these tumours with a striking variety of differenti-ated cell types. So he had the idea that the primordial germ cells were pluripotent, which wasn't a leap, and that they could start to grow and proliferate abnormally and then differentiate.[3]

The two paths did not intersect: the decades of work that led to Thomson's discovery was done in parallel to that of Till and McCulloch's advances in blood-based stem cells, not in combination with it. However, the impact of the discovery of human embryonic stem cells on the public's imagination was profound, triggering mainstream interest in the possibility of growing 'replacement tissues for people with various diseases, including bone marrow for cancer patients, neurons for people with Alzheimer's diseases and pancreatic cells for people with diabetes'.[21] Naturally, it sparked interest into the origins of stem cells and, in so doing, shone a light on the founders of the field of stem cell science: Till and McCulloch (Fig. 14.3).

14.8 Conclusions

Till and McCulloch won the Gairdner Award, Canada's top prize for medical research, and the 2005 Lasker Award. As North America's top prize for health research, the Lasker is frequently the precursor to the Nobel. However, this has not been the case for Till and McCulloch and it now appears their moment truly has passed. With McCulloch's death in 2011 he became ineligible for the prize — it

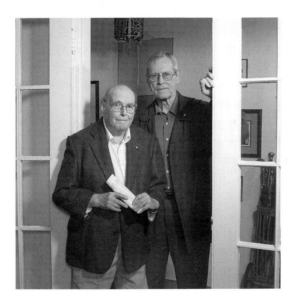

Fig. 14.3. Last photograph taken together, in 2009, with McCulloch holding a copy of their original paper. (Courtesy of Martin Tosoian Photo.)

is only awarded posthumously if the recipient dies after being named a winner. In awarding the 2012 Nobel Prize in Physiology or Medicine to Japan's Shinya Yamanaka for his work on induced pluripotent stem cells — embryonic-like stem cells that are produced by genetically reprogramming mature skin cells — the Nobel Assembly missed a chance to correct a longstanding oversight by including Till as joint winner. Instead they fixed a different but no less glaring oversight, naming the UK's John B. Gurdon, who proved in 1962 that specialization of cells is reversible, as joint winner with Yamanaka. To Till, who has made it clear that winning prestigious awards is 'not why we did this kind of work' and 'not why I went into science',[22] it made good sense. 'The connection between his [Gurdon's] work and Yamanaka's is fairly obvious; they both involve reprogramming DNA in essence.' As to why the Nobel Assembly did not include him, he is characteristically unfazed: 'They had their reasons, I'm sure.'[9]

References

1. Encyclopedia Britannica. *Christopher Columbus.* Available online at: http://www.britannica.com/EBchecked/topic/127070/Christopher-Columbus%20 (Accessed: 28 December 2012).
2. The Lasker Foundation. *Albert Lasker Basic Research Award: Award Description.* Available online at: http://www.laskerfoundation.org/awards/2005_b_description.htm (Accessed: 26 September 2010).
3. Sornberger J. *Dreams & Due Diligence: Till and McCulloch's Stem Cell Discovery and Legacy.* Toronto: University of Toronto Press; 2011.
4. Siminovitch L. *Reflections on a Life in Science.* Toronto: Siminovitch; 2003.
5. Abraham C. Scientist was pioneer in stem cell research. *Globe and Mail,* 29 January 2011; S11.
6. Sask WE. First to make 'cobalt bomb'. *The Leader-Post* (Regina). 28 September 2006; A6.
7. Kraft A. Manhattan Transfer: Lethal Radiation, Bone Marrow Transplantation, and the Birth of Stem Cell Biology, c. 1942–1961 *Historical Studies in the Natural Sciences* 2009; 39: 181–218.

8. Barnes DWH, Ford CE, Gray SM *et al.* Spontaneous and induced changes in cell populations in heavily irradiated mice. *Progress in Nuclear Energy — Biological sciences* 1959; Series 6; Vol 2: 1–10.
9. Interview/email correspondence with the author, November 2012.
10. McCulloch EA. *The Ontario Cancer Institute, Success and Reverses at Sherbourne Street*. Montreal-Kingston: McGill-Queen's University Press; 2003.
11. CBC Radio. *The Current*, 6 December 2011. Available online at: http://www.cbc.ca/thecurrent/episode/2011/12/06/the-story-of-two-canadian-scientists-who-discovered-stem-cells/ (Accessed: 29 December 2012).
12. Google Scholar. Available online at: http://scholar.google.com/schola r?cites=6218129680073699753&as_sdt=2005&sciodt=0,5&hl=en (Accessed: 28 December 2012).
13. Weissman IL. 50 Years Later: Remembering the Paper. *Radiation Research* 2011; 175: 143–144.
14. Becker AJ, McCulloch EA, Till JE. Cytological demonstration of the clonal nature of spleen colonies derived from transplanted mouse marrow cells. *Nature* 1963; 197: 452–454.
15. Siminovitch L, McCulloch EA, Till JE. The distribution of colony-forming cells among spleen colonies. *J Cell Physiol* 1963; 62: 327–336.
16. Till JE, McCulloch EA, Siminovitch L. A Stochastic Model of Stem Cell Proliferation, Based on the Growth of Spleen Colony-Forming Cells. *Proc Nat Acad Sci USA* 1964; 51: 29–36.
17. Trentin JJ. Determination of Bone Marrow Stem Cell Differentiation by Stromal Hemapoietic Inductive Microenvironments. *Am J Path* 1971; 65: 621–628.
18. Wu AM, Till JE, Siminovitch L *et al.* Cytological evidence for a relationship between normal hematopoietic colony-forming cells and cells of the lymphoid system. *J Exp Med* 1968; 127: 455–464.
19. Iscove N. Obituary: Ernest McCulloch. *Cell Stem Cell* 2011; 8: 250–251.
20. Notta F, Doulatov S, Laurenti E *et al.* Isolation of Single Human Hematopoietic Stem Cells Capable of Long-Term Multilineage Engraftment. *Science* 2011; 333: 218–221.

21. Weiss RA. Crucial Human Cell Isolated, Multiplied. *The Washington Post*, 6 November 1998. A01. Available online at: http://www.washingtonpost.com/wp-srv/national/cell110698.htm (Accessed: 28 March 2011).

22. Sornberger JTO. Stem cell pioneers win 'America's Nobel'. *Toronto Star*, 8 September 2005: A8.

Chapter 15

AKIRA ENDO: THE DISCOVERY OF STATINS

Gilbert Thompson and Hiroshi Mabuchi

15.1 Introduction

In his book *Nobel Prizes and Life Sciences*, Erling Norrby[1] provides a glimpse into how Nobel Prize winners are chosen, based on his experiences while on the committee responsible for the prize in Physiology or Medicine. The goal of the selection process 'is to identify contributions representing milestones in the evolution of discoveries in science'. This being so, it is surprising that Akira Endo has not yet been chosen since his discovery in 1976[2] of the first statin, compactin, represented a huge milestone in scientific discovery that has had major implications for the prevention and treatment of atherosclerotic cardiovascular disease. Since then several more statins have been discovered or synthesised and the remarkable ability of these compounds to inhibit hepatic cholesterol synthesis and thus lower serum cholesterol has resulted in them becoming the most commonly used drugs in the world.

15.2 Biography

Akira Endo was born in November 1933 in Akita Prefecture in the northeast of Japan. His war-time childhood was a rather sombre affair but was enlivened by his grandfather who used to take him mushroom picking in the nearby hills, engendering in him a life-long interest in fungi. He excelled in chemistry at high school and managed to get a scholarship to Tohuku University, Sendai, where he studied biotechnology. Immediately after graduating in 1957 he joined the Sankyo Company in Tokyo where his first project as a member of the applied microbiology group was to develop an enzyme preparation that could be used to hydrolyze pectins contaminating wines and ciders. He succeeded in purifying a new pectinase and for this work he was awarded his PhD by Tohoku University in 1966 and a Young Investigator Award in Agricultural Chemistry.

The commercial success of his pectinase provided Endo with the opportunity to study in the United States and he opted to work on lipids at Harvard with Konrad Bloch, who had recently won the Nobel Prize for elucidating the cholesterol biosynthetic pathway. Unfortunately Bloch did not have a vacancy but nevertheless befriended him and encouraged his interest in cholesterol metabolism. Instead, from 1966–1968, Endo did his postdoctoral studies in the Department of Molecular Biology at Albert Einstein College of Medicine, working with Lawrence Rothfield on a phospholipid-requiring enzyme involved in the biosynthesis of bacterial lipopolysaccharide.

While in New York Endo was struck by the high prevalence of coronary heart disease and hypercholesterolaemia in the US, in marked contrast with post-war Japan. On his return there he rejoined Sankyo and in 1971 embarked on a search for a microbial inhibitor of cholesterol biosynthesis. Two years later he discovered compactin, the first inhibitor of hydroxyl methyl glutaryl co-enzyme A (HMG CoA) reductase, the rate-limiting enzyme of cholesterol synthesis, and in collaboration with one of the authors (HM) he subsequently demonstrated its cholesterol-lowering properties in human subjects.

In 1978, Endo left Sankyo for an Associate Professorship in the School of Agriculture of Tokyo University of Agriculture and Technology, where he continued his studies of fungal inhibitors of cholesterol synthesis. He soon discovered monacolin K (lovastatin) and, over the next few years, several other HMG CoA reductase inhibitors. He became a Full Professor in 1986 and retired in 1997. Currently he is a Distinguished Professor Emeritus at Tokyo University of Agriculture and Technology and Director of Biopharm Research Laboratories in Tokyo, where he lives with his wife. His hobbies include hill walking and listening to classical music. He received the Japan Prize in 2006 and the Lasker–DeBakey Clinical Research Award in 2008.

15.3 Cholesterol Metabolism and Coronary Heart Disease in the 1960s

Endo's period of working in New York coincided with a renaissance in lipid research in the US, sparked by the publication of a five-part series of papers in the Medical Progress section of *The New England Journal of Medicine* by Fredrickson *et al.* in 1967.[3] One of the authors (GT) was working in Boston at that time and can still recall the wave of enthusiasm these papers generated among clinicians interested in lipids and cardiovascular disease. Fredrickson's novel classification of hyperlipidaemia drew attention to the role of specific lipoproteins in lipid transport and predisposition to atherosclerosis, the latter being especially severe and premature in patients with hypercholesterolaemia due to an inherited increase in low density lipoprotein (LDL), nowadays known as familial hypercholesterolaemia (FH). The mid-1960s were also the time when serum cholesterol levels and CHD mortality rates reached their respective peaks in the US.[4] It is not surprising therefore that Endo took a keen interest in cholesterol metabolism and that he recognised the therapeutic potential of pharmacological inhibition of cholesterol synthesis.

In 1964, Konrad Bloch and Feodor Lynen were awarded the Nobel Prize in Physiology or Medicine for delineating the multitude of chemical reactions involved in the conversion of acetate to cholesterol. Four years earlier, Marvin Siperstein and M. Joanne Guest[5] had proposed that the site of feedback regulation by cholesterol of its own synthesis was the conversion of HMG CoA to mevalonic acid, a relatively early step on the pathway (Fig. 15.1). Subsequently, Siperstein and Violet Fagan concluded that this feedback involved down regulation of the enzyme responsible for converting HMG CoA to mevalonic acid, namely HMG CoA reductase.[6] All that remained to be done now was for someone to discover a competitive inhibitor of

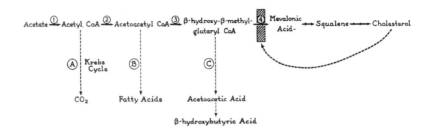

Fig. 15.1. Proposed site of feedback regulation of cholesterol synthesis in 1960. (Reproduced from Siperstein MD and Guest MJ. Studies on the site of the feedback control of cholesterol synthesis. *J Clin Invest* 1960; 39: 642–652, by permission of the American Society for Clinical Investigation.)

this enzyme — which is precisely what Endo aimed to do when he returned to Japan.

15.4 The Discovery of Compactin

Endo has described elsewhere[7] how he and Masao Kuroda started their search for microbial HMG CoA reductase inhibitors after his return to Sankyo in 1971. This was based on the premise that certain microorganisms might produce such compounds as a weapon against competitors dependent for their growth on sterol or isoprenoid metabolites of mevalonate. Inhibiting HMG CoA reductase would prevent synthesis of those metabolites and therefore be lethal to rival organisms.

15.4.1 *In vitro studies*

In order to screen microbial cultures for their ability to inhibit HMG CoA reductase Endo devised a cell-free assay system that measured cholesterol synthesis from ^{14}C-labelled acetate. Over a period of two years he painstakingly screened roughly 6,000 microbial cultures and eventually discovered a strain of *Penicillium citrinum* with inhibitory activity. In July 1973 he isolated the active component from 300 litres of culture medium, ending up with 259 mg of a crystalline compound that was initially named ML-236B but was later called compactin or mevastatin. Compactin inhibited cholesterol synthesis from both acetate and from HMG CoA in nanomolar concentrations but had no effect when mevalonate was used as the substrate. This proved that it was a potent inhibitor of HMG CoA reductase,[2,8] with an affinity for the enzyme that was 10,000-fold greater than the latter's natural substrate, HMG CoA (Fig. 15.2). Using the cultured human fibroblast system devised by Brown and Goldstein for their research on LDL receptors, Endo and colleagues[9] were able to show that compactin was a potent inhibitor of cholesterol synthesis in cells from both a normal subject and a patient with homozygous FH (Fig. 15.3).

By an interesting coincidence workers at Beecham's Laboratories in the UK[10] had independently isolated compactin from *Penicillium brevicompactum* in 1976 while searching for anti-fungal agents. They meticulously described the structure of compactin but its hypocholesterolaemic properties were not investigated at Beecham's until four years later[11] and were then not exploited, which proved to be a lost opportunity in commercial terms.

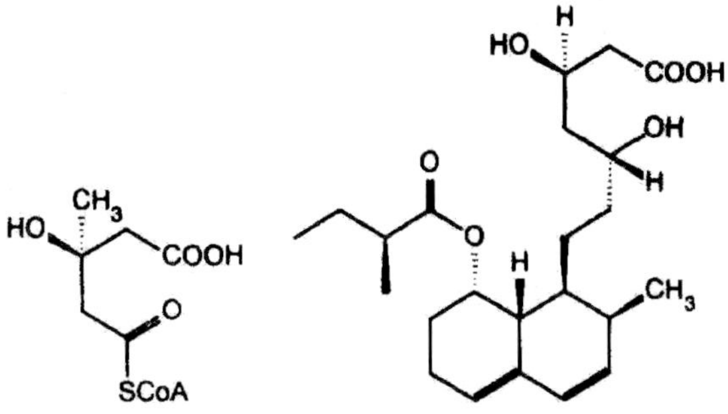

Fig. 15.2. Structural similarity of HMG CoA (left) and the acidic form of compactin (right).

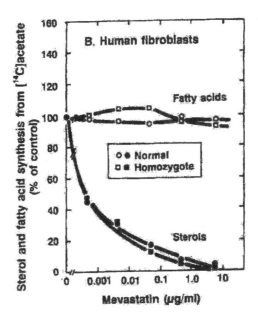

Fig. 15.3.   Inhibition of synthesis of cholesterol but not fatty acids by compactin (mevastatin) in cultured fibroblasts from a normal subject and an FH homozygote. (Modified from Kaneko I, Hazama-Shimada Y and Endo A. Inhibitory effects on lipid metabolism in cultured cells of ML-236B, a potent inhibitor of 3-hydroxy-3-methylglutaryl-coenzyme A reductase. *Eur J Biochem* 1978; 87: 313–321, by permission of John Wiley and Sons.)

15.4.2 *In vivo studies*

Oral administration of single 20 mg/kg doses of compactin to rats acutely reduced their serum cholesterol levels by 20–30%.[2] However, long-term administration to mice and rats was ineffective, probably because the marked compensatory increase in HMG CoA reductase activity that this evoked in the livers of these rodents counteracted the inhibitory effect of compactin.[11,12] In contrast, compactin lowered serum cholesterol by 45% in dogs[13] and also in monkeys, especially reducing their LDL cholesterol.[14]

The first clinical studies with compactin were carried out in 1980 by Akira Yamamoto and Hiroshi Sudo in collaboration with Endo.[15] They showed that compactin doses of 50–150 mg/day reduced serum cholesterol by 27% on average in patients with heterozygous FH or combined hyperlipidaemia, most of the decrease being in LDL cholesterol. Higher doses were needed to lower cholesterol significantly in FH homozygotes, one of whom developed a myopathy which resolved when the dose of compactin was reduced from 500 to 200 mg daily.

The following year one of us (HM) reported the results of administering compactin in a dose of 30–60 mg daily to 7 FH heterozygotes for 24 weeks, which caused a 22% decrease in serum cholesterol.[16] A subsequent study[17] showed that co-administration of the bile acid sequestrant cholestyramine and compactin to FH heterozygotes resulted in an unprecedented 53% reduction in LDL cholesterol after 12 weeks, compared with a 28% reduction when cholestyramine 12 g daily was given alone (Fig. 15.4). Reductions in LDL cholesterol were attributed to stimulation of receptor-mediated LDL catabolism by these compounds, which clearly had an additive effect when given together. In an editorial accompanying the first paper by Mabuchi *et al.*,[16] Brown and Goldstein[18] noted the dramatic reduction in LDL achieved with compactin but cautioned that many hurdles needed to be overcome before it could be regarded as a 'penicillin' for hypercholesterolaemia. The wisdom of this comment soon became apparent when Sankyo suddenly suspended their clinical trial programme, reputedly because of the perceived carcinogenicity of extremely high doses of compactin in dogs (>500 mg/kg/day), and consequently it was never licensed for use in man.

15.5 Other HMG CoA Reductase Inhibitors

Endo had left Sankyo in 1978 to go to Tokyo University of Agriculture and Technology where he continued his studies of fungal inhibitors of cholesterol synthesis. Sankyo had collaborated with the US drug company Merck several years previously by providing them with samples of compactin. The head of research at Merck at the time, Roy Vagelos, had a longstanding interest in HMG CoA reductase and he, like Endo, realised the therapeutic potential of inhibiting this enzyme.

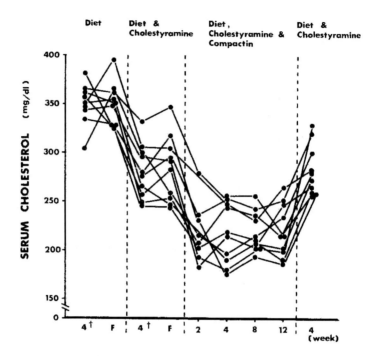

Fig. 15.4.   Effect of cholestyramine alone and in combination with compactin on serum cholesterol in FH heterozygotes. (Reproduced from Mabuchi H, Sakai T, Sakai Y *et al*. Reduction of serum cholesterol in heterozygous patients with familial hypercholesterolemia. *N Eng J Med* 1983; 308: 609–613, by permission of the Massachusetts Medical Society.)

In 1980, his close colleague Alfred Alberts and others at Merck discovered a second HMG CoA reductase inhibitor which they isolated from *Aspergillus terreus*.[19] This was initially called mevinolin but later renamed lovastatin. Endo had isolated the same compound simultaneously but independently from a different mould, naming it monocolin K.[20] He went on to discover several other HMG CoA reductase inhibitors over the next few years before retiring from the university in 1997.

Merck commenced the clinical development of lovastatin but the suspension of all clinical studies on compactin by Sankyo put them in a quandary, especially since Sankyo would not disclose the reason. After much deliberation, as described in detail by Steinberg,[21] Merck followed suit and stopped all clinical work while they undertook additional safety studies in animals. The results were sufficiently reassuring for them to resume clinical trials with lovastatin in 1983. These studies were planned and supervised by Jonathan Tobert, an expatriate clinical pharmacologist from Britain, and four years later lovastatin became the first HMG CoA reductase inhibitor to be licensed by the FDA.[22]

During the interim Merck arranged for lovastatin to be made available to treat patients with refractory familial hypercholesterolaemia on a named patient basis and one of us (GT) and his Hammersmith colleagues gratefully took advantage of this facility from 1983 onwards, with encouraging results.[23] Using radio-labelled LDL, we and others showed that by inhibiting HMG CoA reductase, lovastatin stimulated receptor-mediated LDL catabolism *in vivo*, thereby compensating for the inherent deficiency of LDL receptors in FH patients. The ability to treat these severely hypercholesterolaemic patients effectively and safely with such a well-tolerated compound represented a major therapeutic advance, especially since its LDL-lowering effect of >30% was additive to that of existing therapies such as cholestyramine, partial ileal bypass and apheresis. However, like Yamamoto *et al.*, we found that FH homozygotes were less responsive than heterozygotes. Because of patent constraints lovastatin was never licensed in Britain but Merck maintained supplies for compassionate use until 1989, when its successor simvastatin became available. Simvastatin, a semi-synthetic derivative of lovastatin, differs only in having an additional methyl group which prolongs its duration of action. As will become clear later, it was this compound more than any other which helped to confirm the validity of the lipid hypothesis.

Other statins soon followed, including pravastatin in 1991, which was derived from compactin and developed by Sankyo; fluvastatin in 1994, which was the first synthetic HMG CoA reductase inhibitor; atorvastatin in 1997; rosuvastatin in 2003, the most potent of these compounds and capable of reducing LDL by >50%; and lastly pitavastatin, which was licensed in the US in 2009. Cerivastatin was licensed in 1998 but then withdrawn by its manufacturers on account of its myotoxicity. The latter is the only serious side effect of statins but, cerivastatin apart, is rare with an incidence of <0.1%.[22] The myositis is reversible when the statin is stopped but if left undiagnosed can lead to rhabdomyolysis, renal failure and sometimes death.

The discovery of statins by Endo eventually resulted in huge profits for the pharmaceutical industry but it was not always plain sailing. In addition to early concerns over the suspected toxicity of compactin and the withdrawal of cerivastatin for safety reasons, atorvastatin was nearly scrapped by Parke-Davis on economic grounds. It is said that Roger Newton, who was deeply involved in its development, literally went down on his knees before the Board to plead for its continuation. The directors relented and it became the best-selling drug in the world.

15.6 Statin Trials Resolve the Controversy over the Lipid Hypothesis

As discussed elsewhere,[24] many cardiologists remained unconvinced during the latter part of the 20th century that raised cholesterol caused atherosclerosis or that lowering it by diet or drugs would be an effective means of treating and preventing coronary heart disease. However, those who accepted that cholesterol might play a causal role decided to test this hypothesis by undertaking so-called regression trials, in which the impact of cholesterol-lowering measures on hyperlipidaemic patients with coronary artery disease was assessed angiographically.

The results of a dozen such studies were reported between 1984 and 1994, mostly involving randomised comparisons of diet versus diet combined with lipid-lowering drugs. In the earlier trials bile acid sequestrants were given alone or in combination with nicotinic acid or lovastatin whereas in the later trials lovastatin or simvastatin were given as monotherapy. Angiographic changes were assessed visually or by computer assisted quantitative coronary angiography.

During the trials, LDL cholesterol was 31% lower and HDL cholesterol 5% higher in intervention groups than in controls. Categorisation of patients according to whether their coronary lesions showed angiographic progression, regression, mixed response or no change showed that lipid-lowering therapy reduced progression by one third and increased the chances of regression two-fold. Although not powered to detect changes in clinical endpoints, several trials showed a significant reduction of cardiovascular events in treated subjects.

These trials provided a strong hint that lipid-lowering reduced coronary events but whether it would reduce total mortality was still unresolved. The answer came in 1994 with the publication of the results of the Scandinavian Simvastatin Survival Study (4S), which provided unequivocal evidence that treatment of hypercholesterolae-mia in patients with existing coronary heart disease reduced both cardiovascular events and total mortality.[25] In this epic trial, 4,444 mostly male patients aged 35–70 with angina or previous myocardial infarction and with serum cholesterol averaging 6.8 mmol/l on diet were randomised to receive placebo or simvastatin 20–40 mg/day. During the study, simvastatin reduced total cholesterol by 25%, LDL cholesterol by 35% and increased HDL cholesterol by 8%.

The trial was stopped after 5-and-a-half years because of a highly significant 30% reduction in total mortality in the treatment group, which was due to a 42% reduction in coronary mortality without any change in non-cardiovascular causes of death. In addition, simvastatin significantly reduced the occurrence of cerebrovascular events. The mean level of LDL cholesterol on simvastatin in 4S was 3.2 mmol/l, similar to that in the regression trials. Overall, these findings showed that a 30–35% reduction in LDL cholesterol resulted in decreased progression of coronary atheromatous lesions, fewer clinical events and fewer deaths.

The largest of the statin trials was the Heart Protection Study (HPS),[26] which examined the effects of cholesterol-lowering therapy in more than 20,000 subjects with or at high risk of cardiovascular disease in the UK. Men and women aged 40–80 with serum total cholesterol >3.5 mmol/l were randomised to receive either simvasta-tin 40 mg daily, anti-oxidant vitamins, the two combined or placebo. Subjects on simvastatin had a mean reduction in LDL cholesterol of 1 mmol/l, with decreases in total and cardiovascular mortality of 12%

and 17% and decreases in coronary events and strokes of 26% and 27% respectively. Benefit from simvastatin occurred irrespective of the level of LDL cholesterol at entry to the study, was not influenced by age, gender or clinical status and there was no increase in non-cardiovascular mortality.

The *coup de grâce* for the opponents of the lipid hypothesis came when data from over 90,000 individuals who participated in 14 statin trials between 1994 and 2004 were meta-analysed by the Cholesterol Treatment Trialists' Collaboration.[27] The results were very similar to those in the HPS. Overall, the risk of a major vascular event, including strokes, was reduced by one fifth and no significant changes in non-cardiovascular mortality occurred during five years of statin consumption. Subsequent studies using high doses of more potent statins such as atorvastatin show that the greater the extent of LDL-lowering achieved, the greater the reduction in coronary events and suggest that a 50% decrease in LDL cholesterol could almost halve the risk.

15.7 Role of Statins in Cardiovascular Disease Prevention

Approximately 50 million people are estimated to die in the world each year. In 1990, 28 million deaths were due to non-communicable diseases, more than 10 million of which were caused by coronary heart disease and stroke.[28] The expectation is that by 2020 worldwide mortality from non-communicable diseases will have increased by 80%, with cardiovascular disease remaining as the leading cause of death.[29] Thus it appears that the reduction in cardiovascular mortality occurring in developed countries will be offset by an increase in developing countries, reflecting their adopting the atherogenic Western lifestyle that seems to be an inevitable accompaniment of economic improvement.

It has been estimated that the major modifiable risk factors, namely raised serum cholesterol, smoking and high blood pressure, account for 45%, 29% and 22% respectively of all myocardial infarcts in Western Europe.[30] In England, changes in these risk factors during the past decade have been relatively modest, the prevalence of hypercholesterolaemia in men and women decreasing by 6% and 7.5%, smoking by 14% and 18% and hypertension by 5% and 12% respectively. Changes in the treatment of cardiovascular disease over the same period have been far more marked. Between 1994 and 2005 the number of percutaneous coronary interventions more than tripled, prescriptions for anti-hypertensive and anti-platelet drugs increased four- to five-fold while prescriptions for lipid-regulating drugs, mainly statins, increased by a staggering 2,000%.

In an attempt to explain the 50% decrease in coronary mortality in England and Wales between 1981 and 2000 the number of deaths prevented or postponed by specific cardiac interventions and risk factor changes has been calculated for each of those years.[31] The results suggest that approximately 42% of the decrease was due to cardiological procedures, both medical and surgical, and the remainder to reductions in cardiovascular risk factors. Of the latter, 48% was due to decreased smoking and 10% each to decreases in cholesterol and blood pressure. The large effect of decreased smoking reflects the fact that its prevalence fell by almost 40% during the period under analysis.

A similar study was performed to explain the decrease in coronary mortality in the US over the same period.[32] As in Britain, just under 50% of the reduction in mortality was attributable to medical or surgical interventions and the remainder reflected risk factor changes. In contrast with Britain, decreased smoking accounted for only 12% of the reduction in coronary mortality whereas decreases in serum cholesterol and blood pressure contributed to 24% and 20% of the reduction respectively. The finding that statins made a much larger contribution to the reduction in coronary heart disease mortality in the US than in Britain presumably reflects their longer and greater usage there before 2000.

It is noteworthy that a survey of more than 1,000 patients with FH in the UK showed that their mortality from coronary heart disease had halved since 1992, arguably reflecting the universal use of statins to treat such patients after 1989, when simvastatin was first licensed in Britain.[33] This is supported by data from the Netherlands which shows that statins increased coronary heart disease-free survival among patients with heterozygous FH by 76% and that the risk of myocardial infarction in those over the age of 55 on statins was no greater than that of the Dutch population at large.[34]

Cardiovascular disease and its treatment have an enormous impact on the economy, costing the UK £26 billion a year, 57% of which is direct health care costs.[35] The latter mainly reflect inpatient costs (76%) and medications (18%). Lipid-regulating drugs, mainly statins, cost the National Health Service (NHS) over £600 million in 2005. Currently, about two million people take statins in England and Wales but this is projected to rise to over three million as recent guidelines are increasingly adopted by general practitioners.

There is general acceptance that statin-based strategies for treating and preventing cardiovascular disease are scientifically valid and cost effective in young and middle-aged subjects at high risk,[36–38] especially those with FH. Whether statins should be used across a wider spectrum of ages and risk categories is more contentious. Not only does their cost-efficacy diminish with increasing age but doubts have been cast on the ethics of treating the elderly with these drugs. There is a paucity of evidence that statins reduce total mortality after the age of 70 and, based on the evidence from the Pravastatin in elderly individuals at risk of vascular disease (PROSPER) study,[39] it has been suggested that their use after this age risks substituting a 'less desirable' death from cancer for a 'more desirable' death from coronary heart disease, albeit at a later age. However, there was no increase in cancer deaths in subjects treated with simvastatin in the HPS,[40] although just as many participants in that trial were over the age of 70 as in PROSPER.[39]

Another potential drawback to statin therapy in the elderly is that by reducing mortality from cardiovascular disease it may unintentionally contribute to the rising tide of dementia, especially in those predisposed to both coronary heart disease and Alzheimer's disease by inheritance of apolipoprotein E4. Current evidence suggests that statins reduce mortality in carriers of the ε4 allele but do not protect them against the late onset dementia which accompanies increased longevity.[41]

Despite these caveats, there is little doubt that cholesterol-lowering measures are essential if the premature onset of atherosclerosis and cardiovascular disease are to be prevented at the population level. The downward trend in cardiovascular mortality in the US, Britain and other Western countries suggests that this process is now well under way and underlines the increasingly important role played by statins in modern medicine.

15.8 Conclusions

Having started with an allusion to *Nobel Prizes and Life Sciences* it seems appropriate to conclude with another. In his book[1] Norrby discusses the role of serendipity in science and quotes Pasteur's dictum that 'chance favours the prepared mind'. He gives numerous examples where serendipitous discoveries led to a Nobel Prize, emphasising the importance of determining who first made the critical observation. With regard to the discovery of statins no one disputes Endo's primacy nor would they claim that it was serendipitous. He undoubtedly had a prepared mind but his discovery was certainly not based on chance — he deliberately set out to search for an inhibitor of the key step in the regulation of cholesterol synthesis, using his knowledge of microbiology and lipid biochemistry to pursue this objective.

Mark Twain wrote eloquently about the joys of discovering a new idea, which in Japanese evokes the word '*Ichiban*' or being first. In any language, Akira Endo is one of medicine's pioneers and he deserves due recognition for initiating one of the most important therapeutic advances of recent times. His discovery of the cholesterol-lowering properties of *Penicillium citrinum* more than 35 years ago was as much a first in the treatment of cardiovascular disease as was Alexander Fleming's discovery half a century earlier of the antibiotic properties of *Penicillium notatum* a first in the treatment of bacterial infections. Fleming, together with Chain and Florey, was awarded the Nobel Prize in 1945 for discovering and developing penicillin. Endo, 'whose discovery of statins changed the world' according to Brown and Goldstein,[42] so far lacks such recognition, although he was honoured on this account by the Lasker Foundation in 2008 (Fig.15.5).

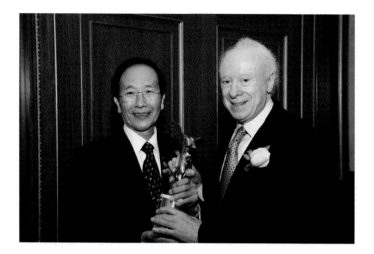

Fig. 15.5.   Akira Endo and Joe Goldstein, Chairman of the Lasker Awards jury and Nobel laureate, after the former received the Lasker–DeBakey Clinical Research Award in 2008.

References

1. Norrby E. *Nobel Prizes and Life Sciences.* Singapore: World Scientific Publishing; 2010.
2. Endo A, Kuroda M, Tsujita Y. ML-236A, ML-236B, and ML-236C, new inhibitors of cholesterologenesis produced by Penicillium Citrinum. *J Antibiotics* 1976; 29: 1346–1348.
3. Fredrickson DS, Levy RI, Lees RS. Fat transport in lipoproteins — an integrated approach to mechanisms and disorders. *New Eng Med* 1967; 276: 34–42, 94–103, 148–156, 215–225, 273–281.
4. Cooper R, Cutler J, Desvigne-Nickens P *et al.* Trends and disparities in coronary heart disease, stroke, and other cardiovascular diseases in the United States. *Circulation* 2000; 102: 3137–3147.
5. Siperstein MD, Guest MJ. Studies on the site of the feedback control of cholesterol synthesis. *J Clin Invest* 1960; 39: 642–652.
6. Siperstein MD, Fagan VM. Feedback control of mevalonate synthesis by dietary cholesterol. *J Biol Chem* 1966; 241: 602–609.
7. Endo A. The discovery and development of HMG-CoA reductase inhibitors. *J Lipid Res* 1992; 33: 1569–1582.

8. Endo A, Kuroda M, Tanzawa K. Competitive inhibition of 3-hydroxy-3-methylglutaryl coenzyme A reductase by ML-236A and ML-236B, fungal metabolites, having hypocholesterolemic activity. *FEBS Lett.* 1976; 72: 323–326.

9. Kaneko I, Hazama-Shimada Y, Endo A. Inhibitory effects on lipid metabolism in cultured cells of ML-236B, a potent inhibitor of 3-hydroxy-3-methylglutaryl-coenzyme-A reductase. *Eur J Biochem* 1978; 87: 313–321.

10. Brown AG, Smale TC, King TJ *et al.* Crystal and molecular structure of compactin, a new antifungal metabolite from *Penicillium brevicompactum. J Chem Soc Perkin 1* 1976: 1165–1170.

11. Fears R, Richards DH, Ferres H. The effect of compactin, a potent inhibitor of 3-hydroxy-3-methylglutaryl coenzyme-A reductase activity, on cholesterologenesis and serum cholesterol levels in rats and chicks. *Atherosclerosis* 1980; 35: 439–449.

12. Endo A, Tsujita Y, Kuroda M *et al.* Effects of ML-236B on cholesterol metabolism in mice and rats: lack of hypocholesterolemic activity in normal animals. *Biochim Biophys Acta* 1979; 575: 266–276.

13. Tsujita Y, Kuroda M, Tanzawa K *et al.* Hypolipidemic effects in dogs of ML-236B, a competitive inhibitor of 3-hydroxy-3-methylglutaryl coenzyme A reductase. *Atherosclerosis* 1979; 32: 307–313.

14. Kuroda M, Tsujita Y, Tanzawa K *et al.* Hypolipidemic effects in monkeys of ML-236B, a competitive inhibitor of 3-hydroxy-3-methylglutaryl coenzyme A reductase. *Lipids* 1979; 14: 585–589.

15. Yamamoto A, Sudo H, Endo A. Therapeutic effects of ML-236B in primary hypercholesterolemia. *Atherosclerosis* 1980; 35: 259–266.

16. Mabuchi H, Haba T, Tatami R *et al.* Effect of an inhibitor of 3-hydroxy-3-methylglutaryl coenzyme A reductase on serum lipoproteins and ubiquinone-10-levels in patients with familial hypercholesterolemia. *N Eng J Med* 1981; 305: 478–482.

17. Mabuchi H, Sakai T, Sakai Y *et al.* Reduction of serum cholesterol in heterozygous patients with familial hypercholesterolemia. *N Eng J Med* 1983; 308: 609–613.

18. Brown MS, Goldstein JL. Lowering plasma cholesterol by raising LDL receptors. *N Eng J Med* 1981; 305: 515–517.

19. Alberts AW, Chen J, Kuron G *et al.* Mevinolin: a highly potent competitive inhibitor of hydroxymethylglutaryl-coenzyme A reductase and a cholesterol-lowering agent. *Proc Natl Acad Sci USA* 1980; 77: 3957–3961.

20. Endo A. Monacolin K, a new hypocholesterolemic agent produced by a *Monascus* species. *J Antibiotics* 1979; 32: 852–854.

21. Steinberg D. An interpretative history of the cholesterol controversy, part V: The discovery of the statins and the end of the controversy. *J Lipid Res* 2006; 47: 1339–1351.

22. Tobert JA. Lovastatin and beyond: the history of the HMG-CoA reductase inhibitors. *Nat Rev Drug Discov* 2003; 2: 517–526.

23. Thompson GR, Ford J, Jenkinson M *et al.* Efficacy of mevinolin as adjuvant therapy for refractory familial hypercholesterolaemia. *QJM* 1986; 60: 803–811.

24. Thompson G. *The Cholesterol Controversy.* London: RSM Press; 2008.

25. Scandinavian Simvastatin Survival Study Group. Randomised trial of cholesterol lowering in 4444 patients with coronary heart disease: the Scandinavian Simvastatin Survival Study (4S). *Lancet* 1994; 344: 1383–1389.

26. Heart Protection Study Collaborative Group. MRC/BHF Heart Protection Study of cholesterol lowering with simvastatin in 20536 high-risk individuals: a randomised placebo-controlled trial. *Lancet* 2002; 360: 7–22.

27. Baigent C, Keech A, Kearney PM *et al.* Efficacy and safety of cholesterol-lowering treatment: prospective meta-analysis of data from 90,056 participants in 14 randomised trials of statins. *Lancet* 2005; 366: 1267–1278.

28. Murray CJ, Lopez AD. Mortality by cause for eight regions of the world: Global Burden of Disease Study. *Lancet* 1997; 349: 1269–1276.

29. Murray CJ, Lopez AD. Alternative projections of mortality and disability by cause 1990–2020: Global Burden of Disease Study. *Lancet* 1997; 349: 1498–1504.

30. Yusuf S, Hawken S, Ounpuu S *et al.* Effect of potentially modifiable risk factors associated with myocardial infarction in 52 countries (the INTERHEART study): case-control study. *Lancet* 2004; 364: 937–952.

31. Unal B, Critchley JA, Capewell S. Explaining the decline in coronary heart disease mortality in England and Wales between 1981 and 2000. *Circulation* 2004; 109: 1101–1107.

32. Ford ES, Ajani UA, Croft JB *et al.* Explaining the decline in U.S. deaths from coronary disease, 1980–2000. *N Eng J Med* 2007;356: 2388–2398.

33. Scientific Steering Committee on behalf of the Simon Broome Register Group. Mortality in treated heterozygous familial hypercholesterolemia: implications for clinical management. *Atherosclerosis* 1999, 142, 105–112.

34. Versmissen J, Oosterveer DM, Yazdanpanah M *et al.* Efficacy of statins in familial hypercholesterolaemia: a long term cohort study. *BMJ* 2008; 337: a2423.

35. Coronary heart disease statistics, 2007 Edition. British Heart Foundation Statistics Database. Available online at: www.heartstats.org (Accessed: 11 July 2012).

36. National Institute for Health and Clinical Excellence. Technology appraisal 94, 2006. Available online at: http://guidance.nice.org.uk/ TA94 (Accessed: 11 July 2012).

37. Pedersen TR, Kjekhus J, Berg K *et al.* Cholesterol lowering and the use of healthcare resources. Results of the Scandinavian Simvastatin Survival Study. *Circulation* 1996; 93: 1796–1802.

38. Mihaylova B, Briggs A, Armitage J *et al.* Cost-effectiveness of simvastatin in people at different levels of vascular disease risk: economic analysis of a randomised trial in 20,536 individuals. *Lancet* 2005; 365: 1779–1785.

39. Shepherd J, Blauw GJ, Murphy MB *et al.* Pravastatin in elderly individuals at risk of vascular disease (PROSPER): a randomised controlled trial. *Lancet* 2002; 360: 1623–1630.

40. Heart Protection Study Collaborative Group. Effects on 11-year mortality and morbidity of lowering LDL cholesterol with simvastatin for about 5 years in 20,536 high-risk individuals: a randomised controlled trial. *Lancet* 2011; 378: 2013–2020.

41. Thompson GR. Cardiovascular disease prevention and the rise in dementia. *QJM* 2012; 105: 93–97.

42. Brown MS, Goldstein JL. A tribute to Akira Endo, discoverer of a 'Penicillin' for cholesterol. *Atheroscler Supp* 2004; 5: 13–16.

INDEX